Dr. Wildlife

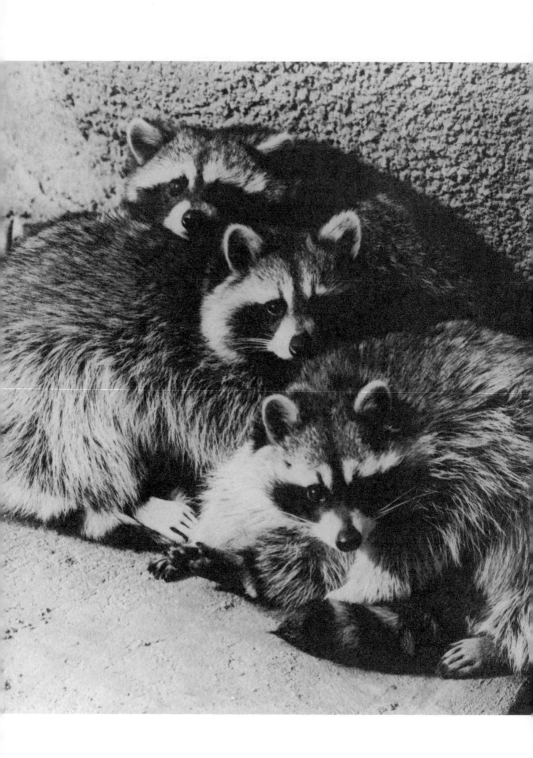

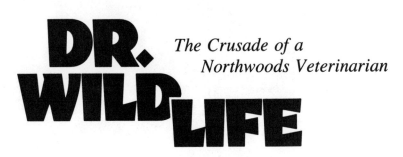

DR. WILDLIFE

*The Crusade of a
Northwoods Veterinarian*

*by Rory C.
Foster, DVM*

*Franklin Watts 1985
New York London*

*The names and identifying characteristics of some of
the individuals and places in this book have been
changed, but the book is autobiographic in scope.*

Library of Congress Cataloging in Publication Data

*Foster, Rory C.
Dr. Wildlife, a Northwoods veterinarian.*

*1. Foster, Rory C.   2. Veterinarians—Wisconsin—
Biography.   3. Wildlife diseases—Treatment—
Wisconsin.   I. Title.
SF996.4.F67   1985   636.089'092'4 [B]   84-22114
ISBN 0-531-09788-9*

*Photographs on frontis and page 164
courtesy of Friends of Animals, Inc.*

To my fishing partners,
  Ali, Michael, and Rori Elizabeth—

But, most of all,
  to my best friend, Linda.

Dr. Wildlife

Acknowledgments

The treatment of injured wildlife and the task of forming a non-profit organization to build a wildlife hospital encompassed the help of many individuals.

For their valuable veterinary expertise and time, I wish to thank the following veterinarians: Dr. Michael Voss, Dr. Thomas Corson, Dr. T. J. Dunn, Jr., Dr. Marty Smith, and my brother, Dr. Race Foster. For his patience and support, I also thank Dr. Pat Redig, Raptor Research Center, University of Minnesota.

Mark Blackburn, perhaps the most knowledgeable avian rehabilitator in Wisconsin, deserves my thanks for his past and continuing support of the project.

John Dunn has been very helpful in many ways, and I'd like to take this opportunity to express my appreciation.

Besides those listed, there have been many, many others who donated time, financial resources, or talent to the wildlife project. For fear of omitting someone, I won't try to list them all. They know who they are and I extend to them my heartfelt thanks.

Carol Ersepke deserves credit for her photographs in the book and on the jacket cover. I'd like to thank her for donating her talents to this book.

For their encouragement and assistance with the manuscript, I thank the following: Gertrude Puelicher, Ted and Beverly Olsen, and Betty Wright. They all helped in their own way with the writing of *Dr. Wildlife*.

And, of course, I thank my wife, Linda, for sticking by me through the tough times and for the warmth and compassion she shared with the patients of the wild.

Rory C. Foster, DVM

Foreword

Many people regard Saint Francis of Assisi as the patron saint of the conservation movement. In his teachings and actions he demonstrated a deep reverence for the lives of all creatures. Christianity and the Western world were thus enriched by the awareness that all creatures are God's handiwork. Consequently, one is morally impelled to respect the divinity within all creatures. This religious view is a forerunner of animal rights philosophy, which holds that all animals have intrinsic worth and are of value to themselves, independent of how we might choose to value or exploit them.

Similarly, Saint Francis of Assisi was in many respects a forerunner of today's conservationists and humanitarians, not all of whom necessarily believe that animals have a "divinity within" or accept animal rights philosophy. Whatever their beliefs are on that subject, however, conservationists are dedicated to alleviating animal suffering, saving endangered species from extinction, and educating the public to conserve natural habitats for wild creatures. Dr. Rory Foster is one of these men.

Here is a veterinarian who has chosen to follow the wisdom of the heart and set up a center where sick and injured wildlife can be treated and rehabilitated, a place that can also serve as an educational resource for the community. That all sounds very wonderful and straightforward, but there are many difficulties in diagnosing and treating the various afflictions and injuries that befall hawks, deer, otters, herons, loons, and other wild creatures. Dr. Foster takes his readers through many case histories, sharing his insight, skills, triumphs, frustrations, and sorrows. A healer is more than a highly skilled technologist, and these vignettes reveal that veterinary medicine is both a science and an art; it requires technical know-how plus the compassion and understanding that are the healer's hallmarks.

Dr. Foster was forced into a political arena in which some people opposed what he was doing. Perhaps the most telling insight in this book is that those governmental authorities in whose trust and responsibility we have placed the lives and welfare of all wild animals frequently violate this trust by shirking their legal and moral responsibilities. The Department of Natural Resources in the state of Wisconsin, for example, actually tried to make it illegal for game species such as deer, beaver, and wild geese to be given first aid or any form of rehabilitative care. Such legislation would have effectively destroyed Dr. Foster's dream of a wildlife hospital and rehabilitation center.

Furthermore, this good veterinarian's accounts of his dealings with some state wildlife officials reveal a common flawed perception of wildlife. They saw no point in treating sick or injured wildlife because the creatures would, after all, be shot by hunters, trapped by trappers, killed by predators, or die from some other natural cause eventually. This rationale is similar to that of the individuals who oppose my advocacy work for humane reforms in "factory" farming of livestock and poultry: Why bother to treat them humanely when they are going to die anyway?

Dr. Foster and others practice the values and virtues of Saint Francis of Assisi both by saving large numbers of animals and by changing the hearts and minds of those who perceive animals as mere things to exploit as they desire. In respecting and treating each animal as an individual, Dr. Foster challenges those who perceive wild animals as harvestable crops; he helps people to see and feel differently: to regard each animal as an individual, with its own intrinsic worth, interests, rights. And in so doing, he brings us all a little closer to appreciating the divinity within each living creature.

Michael W. Fox
Veterinarian and Scientific Director
The Humane Society of the United States
Washington, D.C.

1
Remembrance

It was a sweet spring night in 1982. . . .

My wife Linda and I sat with our backs against a mammoth hundred-year-old white pine, its bark gnarled, which soared upward to a lofty pinnacle etched against a black velvet sky. There a full moon rode high, flooding the courtyard with benign light.

I smiled encouragement at Linda as she tended another car-struck fawn, its brown eyes bright with fear. The fawn had suffered a broken leg, and now Linda was trying to bottle-feed it.

"It'll be all right," I said, trying to reassure her and hoping my voice carried the weight of authority. Sometimes wildlife didn't respond to accepted veterinary practices, and diagnosis was seldom positive and sure. But tonight I was feeling pleased nonetheless. My eyes swung around the courtyard, which encompassed a dream fulfilled.

Before us was the original animal hospital, a building ripe with vivid memories. It was known as the Foster-Smith Animal Hospital, named after its owners—my partner of some two years, Dr. Marty Smith, and me. To our right was a 22-foot hallway connecting our animal hospital to a building that had been completed only a few weeks earlier. Immediately to our left was a 12-foot-high redwood fence connecting the rear of the animal hospital to the new structure behind us, forming the final fixture of the 600-square-foot courtyard in which we sat, its lone feature the old white pine, 150 feet tall, a symbol of countless hours of effort by my partner, my brother, Linda, and me in creating the Northwoods Wildlife Hospital. Here was the first facility in the Midwest built solely for the treatment and care of injured wildlife. The grand opening was scheduled for the very next day, June 19.

I turned to Linda. "Is it my imagination or does this fawn look like Faline?" The spots on the fawn's neck and the contours of her face and ears seemed remarkably similar.

Linda, cradling the fawn like a baby, considered the newborn deer, her face glowing with affection. They were a beautiful sight—the fawn and Linda—beneath the full moon. Finally, Linda shook her head. "I don't know, Rory. The light is playing tricks tonight."

I understood her perfectly. We had raised and released eight fawns since Faline. I laughed, uneasy with my emotions as I reached out and stroked the fawn's smooth coat. "Don't tell me," I said. "I know. All fawns look alike." And I was remembering Faline, how she had been the catalyst for the whole wildlife hospital project, stimulating in me the intense interest in wildlife medicine and surgery that had led to the formation of a nonprofit organization, which in turn, had led to the new wildlife hospital. It had been a long and often frustrating road to travel, but now the future was upon us, and this pleased me.

I glanced upward now at the northern lights, scattering energy with unabashed brilliance over the earth. The immensity of the universe overwhelmed me, but Linda brought me swiftly back to reality.

"Rory," she said urgently, "the fawn's not drinking her milk. I've got to get at least four ounces down her tonight."

I massaged the fawn's smooth neck to produce a swallowing reflex, while Linda held our patient's mouth open with one hand and gently worked the bottle in and out with her other hand. This technique had proven effective in force-feeding fawns in the past.

The fawn began to swallow timidly, taking a bit of much needed nourishment, and I looked into Linda's dedicated and loving face as she fed the fawn. Linda has a gentleness about her that affects me deeply. I knew precisely what I was about when I married her, realizing that someday we would come this way together.

The years since Faline had been busy years for Linda. She

had given birth to our two children, while raising numerous wildlings. But those years didn't show. She was a truly beautiful woman with a lithe and lissome figure. I watched as she leaned over the fawn, encouraging it to drink, her dark hair falling slightly below her shoulders and resting on the fawn's head, her radiant blue eyes filled with sympathy and concern for the fawn. I was touched beyond words. I sat looking at my wife, admiring her, captured by the essence of her. Finally, as if trying to catch up with her, I said quietly, "Is the fawn drinking at all?"

"Not much yet. But she's sucking on her own. That's a good start." She glanced up at me and smiled. "I'll keep trying. We have all night, you know."

She wasn't exaggerating. If it took all night to get the fawn to drink, Linda would do it. "Compassion," I sometimes told her, "is your profession." Always she would laugh in response, as if I made no sense at all. But it was true.

I liked to think that I was moved by the same compassion. But I understood that part of my commitment was rooted in my professional training and a natural desire to turn learned skills into practical application. I was expected to care. It was that simple. But Linda's motives were uncomplicated by veterinary degrees and oaths. She truly loved her work with animals. Whether the patient was a graceful fawn or a tiny, defenseless robin, I could count on Linda. She stood by me always, ever helpful and eager to assist and please.

Now she was saying, "Can you believe it, Rory?"

"Tomorrow?"

"Yes, tomorrow morning at nine o'clock."

"It's hard to believe," I admitted.

"Amazing, huh?"

"Especially after everything that's happened . . ." Surprisingly our concept of treating wildlife for eventual release into the forest had created a disturbing and negative response in the north woods—indeed throughout the state of Wisconsin.

One local resident had claimed in a letter to the newspaper, "It would be better to salvage the meat and hide" from our patients than to give them a helping hand. That opinion was echoed by many other people. We had fought a year-long public debate on the subject of treating injured wild creatures, though we had solicited no public funds. My partner and I along with other members of our wildlife organization were footing the bill for this care, and we couldn't understand the opposition.

Perhaps the most shocking opposition came from state institutions that supposedly existed to protect wildlife—in particular, the Wisconsin Department of Natural Resources. Time after time this agency and its employees fought our efforts to establish the hospital. At one point, the agency proposed state legislation that would make it illegal to help some injured wild animals. Only after a lengthy, bitter campaign by my partner and me was the proposed legislation dropped. It seemed totally illogical that we should have been forced to publicly defend our position and justify our aim to help wild creatures. We had begun with the very best of motives, and we were sincere in what we did.

After Faline had come into our lives, I had begun accepting more and more wildlife patients. Along came an injured hawk, then a loon and an owl. Treating them seemed natural and right.

Soon our animal hospital became known in our area as the sanctuary for injured wild creatures of all kinds. It became obvious to us that if we were to continue this work, we would need a larger and more specialized facility to accommodate these patients and treat them properly.

True, the existing hospital was modern and well equipped. In fact, I prided myself on one point especially; it was one of only a handful of small animal hospitals in Wisconsin to receive certification by the American Animal Hospital Association, an organization of elite dog and cat hospitals that spoke of the highest standards in veterinary medicine. But as functional and pleasant as it was, it did not have the facilities for wildlife.

The dogs and cats, not to mention the constant flow of human traffic in our building, were not conducive to good healing in testy great horned owls and fractious goshawks. Even the white-tailed deer, a relatively adaptable species, didn't take well to the clinic. That's why, five years earlier, Linda and I had raised Faline in our home. But the real difficulty hadn't been the uproar of public debate about the concept of treating injured animals, or even the events that led to the building of the wildlife hospital. The real challenge, at least for me, was to become competent in wildlife veterinary practice, not an easy knowledge to acquire.

Most definitely this knowledge was not conferred on me by my undergraduate zoology degree or by my four years of veterinary medical school. There was no residency in wildlife medicine and surgery. And so, I began what might be called a self-apprenticeship, a period of several years in which I studied wildlife anatomy and physiology, collaborating with known experts in the field, while learning to apply the basic veterinary skills I had already mastered to new and different species. Exactly when that apprenticeship will end is hard to say, since I'm learning still. But nowadays I feel a certain competency that I did not possess in earlier days, and I sense I'm well on my way.

When an injured hawk comes in, I don't have to retreat to the back office to verify the species or check the dosage of anesthetic needed for surgery. I can look at an X-ray and determine at a glance if a loon's shattered wing is mendable by surgery; if it is, I know the procedure to follow. In other words, I no longer experience that sinking feeling of helplessness in the gut when I'm presented with a badly injured wild patient—and this tells me I'm doing well. At this point a certain joy comes over me, the elation of personal satisfaction, which has nothing to do with congratulatory letters of proclamations from an approving veterinary board.

To be sure, some recognition has been given me. Colleagues call for advice or refer patients to me for treatment. Others hear of my work and send words of encouragement. But the greatest rewards come directly from the wild patients—as a majestic bald eagle flies free after a close brush with death; or when an owl rises upward, its wing mended, never to return to

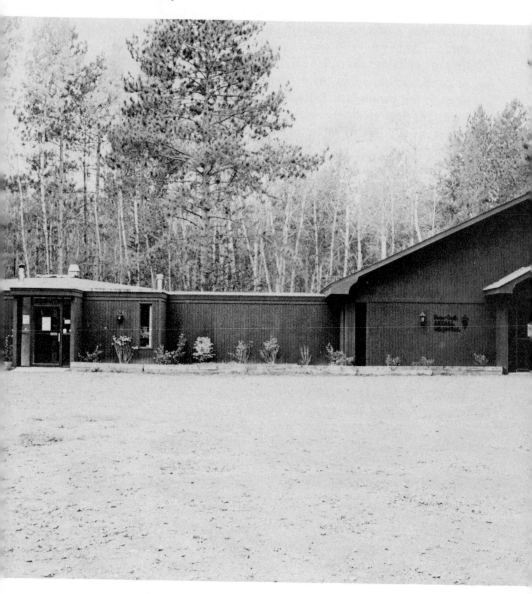

The Northwoods Wildlife Hospital

confinement; or on the day that a fawn, its leg healed at last, flicks its tail in a jaunty salute and disappears into the green wilderness. These are the true rewards, the ones that never diminish. They are there always, fond memories that exalt the spirit. . . .

"How's it going, Linda?" I reached out and stroked the fawn.

"Slow," she murmured. "It may take a while."

"There's no hurry," I told her. "It's pleasant here tonight."

"And very special," she said.

Yes, so special that I felt no need to hurry home to bed. I settled in comfortably, my back against the old tree. A veil of tranquillity hung shimmering in the air, a fitting calm before the next day's activities.

Several television crews would be there for the opening of the Northwoods Wildlife Hospital. Many of Wisconsin's leading newspapers would send reporters to cover the event. Despite the promised publicity, I wasn't looking forward to the festivities. The opening was newsworthy, to be sure, and public relations were important, but it seemed to me that these events were incidental to the real story, which was unfolding now—tonight and right here with the injured fawn.

A week earlier, we had rescued an orphaned long-eared owl. And, yes, a week before that, we had operated on a loon, removing a fishhook from its stomach. No, I thought, the real story wouldn't be captured on film tomorrow or recounted by a newspaper reporter as the doors opened to the new hospital.

The crisp night air invaded my jacket. I zipped it up and moved closer to Linda, resting my head against the familiar old tree. Linda, too, snuggled nearer, her head on my shoulder as she continued to feed the fawn.

Tomorrow wasn't the beginning of the story. The story had begun with Faline. And my mind drifted back, remembering. . . .

2 *And Don't Forget to Make Your Bed*

Faline wasn't a very original name for a deer, but that's the name Linda picked for the first fawn we ever raised. She chose the name because Walt Disney's *Bambi* had made a lasting impression on her in early childhood, and she'd always had a soft spot for anything small and helpless. I'm sure the lack of originality was also due to the suddenness with which the tiny fawn entered our lives.

Early one morning in late May a motorist had discovered her lying next to the highway. He had carefully transported the injured fawn to the nearest animal hospital—my facility in Minocqua, Wisconsin.

The motorist was a man of about sixty with a tanned and pleasant face. His bushy gray hair peeked out from under a white fishing cap with trout streamers hooked onto the front. Underneath his chest-high waders, he wore a khaki fishing vest, which bulged with fishing accessories. On the front of the vest was a small hairlike patch with more trout flies attached. As he came through the front door of the hospital, the patch on his vest reminded Linda of a miniature launching pad armed with tiny missiles for battling wily brook trout; evidently the extra seconds needed for deployment from a concealed pocket could be critical. Every necessity had to be there in front, ready and waiting at just the right time.

He said to Linda, who worked as my receptionist, "Excuse me, miss, but do you take care of injured fawns here?"

Linda considered, but only briefly. "Well, sure. Why not?"

I came in then, having overheard the short conversation, but Linda plunged onward, determinedly. "I'll need a little information, though, for our records." She placed a pen and a patient information sheet before her on the desk. "Now, let's see. What's the fawn's name, and how old is she?"

The man's eyes were puzzled. "Well, now, you don't seem to understand. She's not my fawn. I found her on the road to my fishin' hole. She's not mine."

"Oh?" said Linda. "I thought she was probably yours. Some people in this area have pet deer. Anyway, don't worry. I'll get Dr. Foster." She turned, and there I was. "This man has an injured fawn, and I think we should do something right away." Linda's dark eyes danced with excitement.

I smiled at her. "Maybe we'd better have a look at it. Where is it?" I asked the fisherman.

"In my Chevy Blazer out front." He led the way outside, where I found a fragile-looking fawn in the back of the man's vehicle.

"This is how I found her, Doc—just a few miles down the road." He pointed west along Highway 70, the road that ran in front of the hospital. "I was on my way trout fishin', and the car in front of me hit her. But the son of a bitch didn't stop. I'm not one of these wildlife freaks—I hunt deer—but I just couldn't keep on going."

"Oh . . ." Linda murmured and leaned forward for a closer look at the fawn.

His words had touched me, too. He gave credibility to my own privately held theory that most trout fishermen are true sportsmen; they seem to appreciate wildlife more than most.

"She needs help," I ventured. "That's plain to see." Then, I lifted the fawn gently from the Blazer.

The fisherman climbed into the driver's seat of his vehicle. "Well," he called out, as he started the engine, "I sure hope you can help her, Doc. I just couldn't leave her."

I nodded understanding as he drove away with a wave of his hand.

Linda and I returned to the hospital where I placed the small trembling fawn—its legs bent and much too long and bony for the speckled velvet body—on the examining table. I felt the fawn's heart beating wildly, and I saw the terror in the soft doe's eyes.

Suddenly, unexpectedly, I was hearing that familiar alarm inside me, the alarm I had not experienced since graduation from veterinary school, when I felt sometimes less than confident. In my two and a half years of practice, I thought this alarm had been laid to rest once and for all time. Not so. The question was: Could I help this small fragile creature in distress?

I was accustomed to the sight of newborn domestic animals, but this was the first time I had seen a newborn white-tailed deer. The umbilical cord was withered but still attached. I guessed the fawn to be about forty-eight hours old, and she weighed a mere four and a half pounds. Her moist black nose nuzzled urgently against my palm, as if she might be looking for a familiar smell of reassurance. Delicately, oh, so carefully, I began to examine her.

On her head were two abrasions covered with clotted blood. A minor laceration creased her lower lip. No serious head injuries, I thought, since the large, dark eyes were clear and symmetrical. Her ears flicked continuously in all directions as she explored this strange new world. "Her hearing's fine," I ventured.

Linda nodded, her eyes seeking more reassurance.

I couldn't give it. The grating of bone in the fawn's left hip signaled a fracture. Radiographs substantiated this diagnosis. She had sustained a fracture of the femur, and the small size of her body prevented her from walking on her three good legs. If the trout fisherman had left her beside the highway, she would have died.

"We'll keep her comfortable," I told Linda. "Tonight we'll do surgery."

Throughout the remainder of the day, when Linda had a break from caring for our dog and cat patients, she tended the fawn, cleaning the head wounds with hydrogen peroxide and applying an antiseptic ointment. Already Linda was calling the fawn Faline, smiling at me as she did, explaining herself lightly. But I knew within my heart that something special was happening here as I administered antibiotics to lessen the chances of bone infection following the surgery that would be necessary to repair the leg.

Once the doors of the hospital were closed, we became very busy. While Linda monitored the anesthetic, I set about reducing the fracture. I placed two stainless-steel pins along the length of the femur to hold the broken segments in proper alignment to ensure good healing. Later, when the break was healed, I would remove the pins.

I had taken every precaution; I had done my best. Now all we could do was watch and wait.

Linda sat with the fawn, stroking her golden coat, which was covered by splotches of white like a late spring snow, camouflage against predators. Now and then she turned the fawn to hasten its recovery. "I don't know," she said over and over. "It's taking an awfully long time for her to wake up."

I paced the floor, doing little odds and ends around the hospital. "Give her time."

The waiting seemed to go on forever. Finally, two long hours later, Faline began to stir.

"Oh, Rory, look!" Linda was excited. "She's coming around!"

Faline sat up and looked at us with those very large and beautiful brown eyes.

"I think she's going to be okay," I said. "But there'll be a long recovery."

"We don't have a place for her here. Could we—could we—"

I knew what Linda was trying to ask me. "Take her home?"
"Yes."

I relented easily. "She'd be frightened and lonely here."
"She's come to know us now."

"Yes. That's why we should take her home. Anyway, I won't turn her over to one of the game farms."

"Oh, no," Linda said. "They'd keep her forever in captivity."

"That's for sure. But remember. It's going to be a great deal of work. She's awfully young. Anything can happen. Try not to get too attached to her."

I didn't want to sound pessimistic, but I knew that raising injured wild animals from an early stage was seldom easy; inevitably some died. Meanwhile, though, I knew that cautioning Linda about becoming emotionally involved was like whistling in the wind. Her vulnerability with homeless puppies and kittens had been demonstrated countless times in the past. And so it was to be with Faline.

From that night on, Linda took over the fawn. She was up every four hours day and night. Linda was Mother Earth and I loved her for it. Her spindly little charge Faline loved her, too. I could see the rapport grow between them as Linda poked and prodded vitamins down Faline's slender throat, administered antibiotics on a regular schedule, fed Faline from a bottle for long hours, and devised physical therapy to improve the fawn's muscle strength through massage.

Noting on occasion how tired Linda looked, I offered my help.

"No, thanks, Rory. Faline has grown accustomed to my touch."

I let it be, smiling to myself. What else could I do? Linda's efforts were paying dividends. The fawn was recovering nicely, and I was proud of Linda as Faline stood for the first time and took her first tentative steps.

As the weeks passed, Linda and Faline became more and more entranced with each other. The fawn knew the instant Linda entered the yard. When Linda knelt, holding out her arms, Faline came to her as fast as she could, wobbly though she was, full of affection for this gentle friend who had helped to make her well again. But it didn't end here. They touched noses and nuzzled, while Faline's small white tail flicked like a flag. The fawn had become a member of the family.

By July Faline's fracture had healed, and I removed the pins from her leg. We no longer had an excuse for keeping Faline confined. We gave her the freedom to come and go. At night Faline preferred to sleep in the woods near our home. But during the day she spent several hours with our family.

At that time, besides Linda and me, the family included Tenille, a golden retriever whose beauty was matched by intelligence and breeding. She was a big dog, but she was unusually gentle with smaller animals, especially if they were hurt. The other member of the family was the cat, Billy Finn.

His name was pinned on him because his hair resembled one of my old fishing lures. It was called a Billy Finn bucktail. Both had long extravagant hair, partly black and the rest pure white. Billy Finn was a large cat and, like an Irishman, he had an easy manner but he was a tough fighter if backed into a corner. And, he was loyal and true to those he looked on with favor. Billy Finn was a fine gentleman cat.

With Billy Finn, Tenille, and now Faline, we had a full house. But it was all great fun, and nobody enjoyed it more than Linda.

Throughout the summer, the camaraderie that developed between Linda and Faline was truly special. Linda thought of Faline as her first child, and, of course, she had nurtured the fawn like an infant. They played, walked in the woods, nuzzled or sat quietly side by side, feeling and knowing that what was between them was good and trusting and lasting.

As summer matured into early autumn, Faline's body began to change, too. She filled out, and nature's protection, her spots, faded rapidly. She weighed sixty pounds now, and her natural instincts began to manifest themselves.

The author's wife, Linda,
and Faline

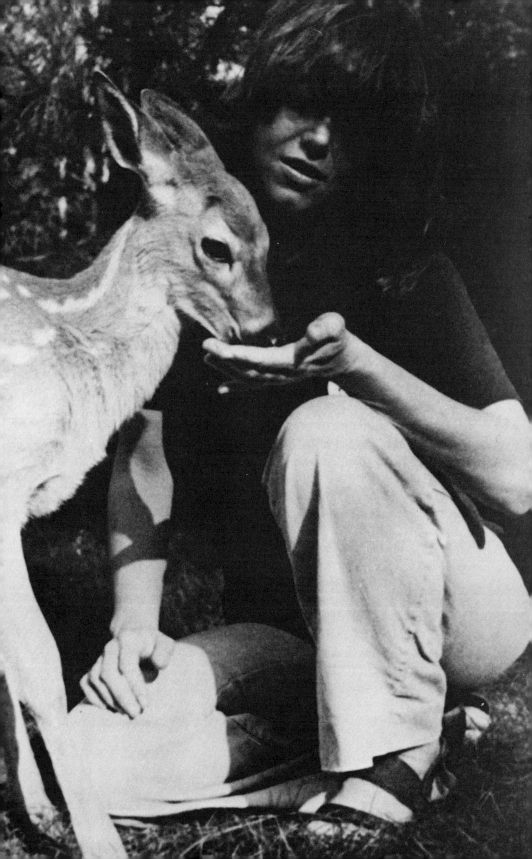

One night after we were in bed, Linda said into the darkness, "Faline has a distant look these days. I think I'm losing my child." Her voice was wistful for good things quickly passing.

"You knew this day would come," I reminded her, but not too forcefully. I didn't want to hurt her any more than she was about to be hurt.

"I know, I know. But it's too soon."

I had been putting this moment off. But now it had to come. "I think we should release her somewhere far away from here. We're too near the highway. It's only a half-mile, and I—"

"But," Linda protested, "Can we take her where she'll be perfectly safe? I mean—"

"I know what you mean, but, Linda, nowhere is perfectly safe. The time's come. Faline's eating on her own. Her leg is sound."

"She deserves to be free," Linda agreed.

"Of course she does. How about that place down by the trout stream. It's at least five miles from the nearest main road or house. I'm sure she'll be safe there."

Linda didn't answer. She knew as well as I did that no place was truly safe for Faline in the woods. And so we fell asleep one more night, putting off the decision on freeing Faline. We had come to care too much, and we both knew it.

Days of procrastination passed. Finally, we came to grips with the subject again. This time we could not put it off. It was up to us to give Faline her freedom, and she deserved it now.

On a late September day with the falling of leaves and the ripple of rain, we led Faline into the Bronco and set off through the autumn of red and gold and orange to freedom. Neither of us spoke. It was a day we would not forget.

Because Faline disliked small places and confinement, I had administered a mild, short-acting sedative to facilitate the drive to the woods. She took the trip well, and I knew the drug-induced sleep would last only ten minutes or so after we arrived.

I lifted Faline from the Bronco, and Linda and I sat down,

our backs against a small white birch tree, holding Faline close to us, while we waited those last minutes for the sedative to wear away. I glanced at Linda.

Tears streamed down her face to fall silently on the silken head pressed close to her body. Watching her caress Faline and knowing the ache in her heart, I felt as if I might cry, too. It was time to give up Faline, but doing it wasn't easy.

Now Faline would have to make it on her own. Both Linda and I were worried. How could we possibly teach her to watch out for poachers? How could we warn her not to trust other human beings as she had trusted us? Would she be able to detect the scent of a predator? Would she find high ground before falling victim to deep snows? And there was the killer highway. The list of fears bombarded our minds. All we could do was give her the chance to try. . . . And I was remembering another September day all too well.

It was in the late 1960s. My parents were dropping me off at a large college campus to begin my education. After we had hugged for the last time, I turned toward my dormitory and saw that my mother was crying, saying, "I'll never see my child again!"

Of course, no such thing had happened. She had seen me often since that day. But to her mind the boy was gone forever.

I recollected stopping halfway up the walk to my dorm and looking back to wave. Mother called after me, "Don't forget to make your bed, Rory."

I nodded casual agreement and turned away. As I climbed the steps to my dorm room, I felt disappointment. I had imagined some profound statement would send me along the road to my future in good form. Instead I had received "Don't forget to make your bed."

My mother's words had seemed silly, incongruous. But now, a decade later, they seemed precise and right. My mother had understood that it was too late for counsel or advice. The matter was out of her hands.

Suddenly and without warning, Faline awakened and leaped

from Linda's lap. She paused just long enough for Linda to give her one last hug of farewell. Then she bounded playfully away from us, pausing here and there to sniff the swirling winds of autumn. Soon she approached the top of a little knoll. She turned and glanced back as if to acknowledge our final parting. Unexpectedly the sun slashed through the birch trees as the day cleared to reflect Faline in all her golden splendor, beautiful and free at last.

I wanted to yell after her, "Don't go, Faline. Don't go." Instead I called out, "And don't forget to make your bed!"

Faline's large velvet-brown eyes touched us for a brief instant of love; then she twitched her tail and was gone.

Linda glanced over at me but didn't question my departing remark. It's a good thing too because I don't think I could've said another word.

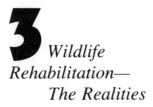
3 *Wildlife
Rehabilitation—
The Realities*

In those first months after Faline came into our lives, I began
treating more and more injured wild patients. I read every book
I could find that related to wildlife care and rehabilitation. I re-
freshed my memory of comparative anatomy and physiology.
Species identification of avian patients was the most difficult
subject; I pressed Petersen's *Field Guide to Birds* into active duty,
shoving it into my hip pocket, where it remained handy. Meanwhile, I learned that restraining birds of prey was hazardous duty.
I mastered the technique only after I had felt talons stab through
my index finger four times!

None of this, though, was as troublesome as coming to terms
with the realization that many of my patients would never be
released to live free again in the wild. This was so disheartening
to me that I began to investigate wildlife rehabilitation organizations.

I learned that only about half of the wild patients treated
were ever released. The other half either died during treatment
or their injuries left them so crippled they were unable to live in
the wild again.

The low success rate, of course, resulted from the severity
of many of the injuries. Fully three-fourths of them were trauma
victims—injured by automobiles or guns—and had suffered broken bones and internal injuries of the worst sort. Further, the
paucity of qualified treatment centers, and the often great dis-
tances involved between accident victim and competent doctor,
took an added toll. All in all, it was not an encouraging picture.

The first screech owl I treated was a good example of the
problems we faced. The owl had been hit by a car near Green

Bay, Wisconsin, and had suffered a compound fracture of the humerus. A full seventy-two hours passed before it arrived at my hospital in Minocqua. During this time, the two-inch segment of bone protruding through the skin had devitalized and effectively died. Had the time lapse between injury and treatment not been so great, the owl might have healed nicely. But such was not the case, and sadly so.

Occasionally the delay was even longer. One of the first loons I treated came to my clinic on a cold and dreary November day, after it was discovered sitting on a frozen lake. As always, I was quite taken by this water bird, which is the size of a goose, long-bodied, with a thick, pointed bill.

Loons are known for their wild laugh and mournful yodel at dusk and during the night. Expert divers all, they plunge as deep as two hundred feet in search of food. In the water they go unmatched, but on land they propel themselves forward on their breasts, and they do this with great difficulty. Already the loon in question had its winter coloring—gray in the crown, hind neck, and underparts, with a white throat. It was ready for winter. But was I ready for the loon?

Radiographs revealed a fracture and dislocation of the right elbow. The injuries had to have occurred at least three months earlier. Since the loon could swim and eat, it had managed to survive until the lakes froze. I wanted to weep for this beautiful creature for now there was nothing that could be done to help it fly.

Learning to cope with hopelessness was frustrating and depressing. I tried to put it out of my mind. It didn't work. While my enthusiasm for what I was doing was maintained, I couldn't help addressing the issue in the back of my mind constantly. Orville, the seagull, was a perfect case in point.

"This is Orville," said the blue-eyed blonde from Ashland College as she set a cardboard box on the reception counter at the hospital. "I was walking along the beach on Lake Superior collecting crustaceans for my marine biology class, and I found him sitting on a rock. Seagulls weren't on my list of specimens, but I picked him up anyway. I named him after my grandfather. He loved birds.''

I looked into the box and considered the seagull. ''Orville, huh? Did he try to fly when you approached him? Did you notice any evidence of injury or anything unusual?'' I tried to get every tidbit of information possible. Sometimes human observations were critical in establishing a cause of injury and assisted in the diagnosis.

''No,'' said the coed. ''He didn't try to fly at all. He just sat there looking lonely and hungry. It was almost as if he wanted me to pick him up. I got some minnows from my brother's bait shop. He ate four. Then I called the local vet. He told me to bring him here. This is the right place, isn't it? It took nearly two hours to get here.''

I smiled wryly. ''Yeah, this is the right place. I'll take care of him. I hospitalize patients like Orville for examination and observation. Usually I take X-rays to search for injuries that may not seem obvious, and I do other tests, if necessary. Does that sound all right to you?''

The girl appeared to be a bit nervous, her bright blue eyes drifting away from mine. ''That sounds good. But I have to tell you—I have to tell you that I can't pay for it all at once. Do you do billing here?''

''Yes, we do allow spread-out payments. But not in this case.'' A flash of panic crossed her face. I smiled to alleviate her worries. ''There's no charge.''

''No charge?'' Her pert young face took on hope.

''That's right. Helping wild animals is my hobby.''

I enjoyed telling people that I treated wildlife for free. The harsh economic realities of veterinary medicine are a great pitfall to small-animal practice, to my way of thinking. Being told not to do a needed laboratory test or surgical procedure because the owner can't afford the expense is something with which every vet must live. So I just avoided the whole business of money in my wildlife practice. I paid for it myself; it became my hobby. In this manner there was never any discussion necessary to jus-

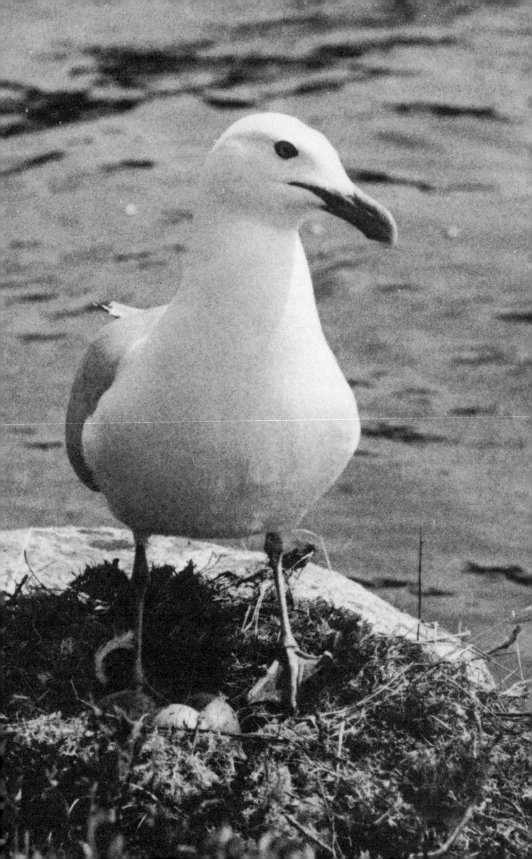

tify X-rays or blood tests, and no lengthy consultations with an owner. If a wild patient needed something, I did it.

Now the pert blonde stepped back and eyed me cautiously. "You mean—there's no charge?"

"No charge at all. Just leave Orville with me, and I'll do my best."

"That's nice," she said softly. "Really nice. If there's anything else I can do, just let me know. Once Orville's better, I'll pick him up and drive him out to Lake Superior."

I laughed. "If he gets better, he can fly back himself. But thanks just the same."

The idea of Orville flying home on his own was an image the girl enjoyed. Relieved and happy, she departed the hospital, waving all the way.

I carried the box back to the treatment room. Orville peered curiously around, putting up no fuss at all. I reached into the box and picked him up gently, placing him on the prep table. His slate-gray wings with black tips were folded neatly against his light gray body, but he bobbed slightly up and down as he tried to secure footing on the shiny stainless steel surface of the prep table.

This was my first seagull. But the plan of attack I'd outlined to the girl seemed logical enough. Carefully I went over Orville with my hands, searching for any irregularities. Fish-line wounds around wings and fishhooks embedded in tissue are common problems in water birds. Orville had none. His eyes were normal. I pried open the beak. No clue there either. Strange, I thought; something's wrong. Certainly no seagull I had ever seen would sit so quietly and willingly on a prep table!

I was on the verge of scooping Orville up in the palm of my hand to head for the X-ray room when I noticed a just dis-

A proud seagull guards her nest
on the shores of Lake Superior.

cernible bulge in the feathers on the left side at the base of his tail. I smoothed the area with my hand and took another look. Sure enough, the feathers there rose slightly above the rest. Parting the deep, long primary quills, I discovered a grape-sized growth protruding from the skin. It was an angry cherry-red lesion. I hesitated. I didn't want to hurt Orville, but it was necessary to palpate the area. Orville didn't mind. The bump was only part of the problem; I could feel the mass was well entrenched in the underlying muscles. Evidently, this thing, whatever it was, interfered with Orville's muscle control of his tail feathers. No wonder he couldn't fly. But what was it?

My mind ranged far and wide. Perhaps there was a pellet from a BB gun or a fishhook embedded deeply in the skin. Just, perhaps, it was really that simple. So, it was off to the X-ray room. The pictures told the story: Orville had a slightly less than golfball-sized mass, most of it located deep in the tail region.

Diagnostically the next step was to do a biopsy on the mass or try to remove it entirely. But first, I needed three days in which to build up Orville for the surgery. I fed him large quantities of minnows along with vitamins and minerals. Three days later, on schedule, Karen, my newly graduated technician, and I set to work on Orville's surgery.

"Is he breathing all right?" I asked Karen.

"Rapid," said Karen, "but okay, I think. It's hard to tell with the machine."

Karen was referring to the oxygen bag on the gas anesthetic machine. Normally, when an anesthetized animal breathes, the bag can be seen expanding on exhalation and contracting during inhalation. But Orville was a twenty-ounce seagull, and his lung capacity was so small that the bag barely moved.

Now with the surrounding feathers pulled back and the skin cleaned and disinfected, I placed a surgical drape over and around the mass and began to cut. The dissection to remove the growth was slow and delicate, terribly tedious, but I was doing well, and there was not much bleeding. When I got near the base, however, things became a bit more tough. Tentaclelike roots from the mass invaded the glistening muscles below. With each snip of the dissecting scissors, more bleeding occurred.

After nearly an hour, I had removed as much of the growth as possible. I wasn't sure I had gotten it all, but to go farther into Orville's body would have meant certain loss of muscle and nerve control. So I chose to go no deeper. I wanted Orville to fly again. Success in Orville's case hung on more than just removing the invading growth. I was gambling, hoping I had removed the problem while leaving vital control areas of the tail feathers intact.

Almost done now, I said to Karen, "Turn the anesthetic off and give only oxygen."

Karen eyed the bloody mass of tissue laying on the table beside Orville. "What do you think it is?"

"Cancer," I murmured forlornly.

"I didn't know birds could get cancer."

"Birds," I told her unhappily, "have a higher rate of malignant cancer than any other vertebrate—and that includes humans." It never ceased to amaze me how many common denominators there are in all of life's forms. Cancer was but one of them.

Orville recovered nicely. Later that day, he ate and appeared to be back to normal. But eleven days later, when I received the pathology report, "Fibrosarcoma, guarded prognosis," my optimism vanished. Well, I thought, the only hope was that it might not recur.

Throughout the next three weeks, Orville and I developed a special kinship. I spent extra time giving him his daily exercise, and I fed him myself instead of delegating the task to others. Meanwhile, more than frequently, I checked the surgery site for signs of regrowth. And thirty-three days after Orville's surgery, I could detect a new firmness in the tail region where the original tumor had been excised. I hoped it was my imagination, but four days later, there was no doubt about it. The cancer was at work again, growing, and it seemed to be deeper than before.

Convinced that Orville was doomed, I considered putting him to sleep humanely. Then I looked at Orville overall rather than at the site of the cancer. Orville didn't appear to be suffering. He was alert and eating well.

"No," I told Orville firmly, "We're going to see this one through together."

Though the statistics were against me—one in two thousand—that Orville might undergo spontaneous regression of the malignant growth, I wanted to will him to get well. It was important both to Orville and to me.

For another four weeks Orville was bright-eyed and chipper. During this time, many visitors to the hospital who saw him as a cancer victim came to realize something of that common fabric in all life that binds us closer together as God's living creatures and spills over into the mind. Life at best is a terminal condition; we all must die. So what matters most is how life is lived. And Orville was indeed living life to the fullest.

Each day I allowed him to sit in the treatment room where he could monitor the clinic's activity. Orville would call out, "Kee-ow, kee-ow," at the dogs he loved to tease. In the evenings, when I worked late, Orville sat on my desk to scrutinize my paperwork. Then, along came August.

I arrived at the hospital one morning to have Karen tell me, "I think Orville's getting worse. His feathers seem ruffled, and his eyes are dull. He hasn't been squawking and squealing as he usually does every morning."

With a sense of dread for my companion, I hurried back to Orville's cage. His eyes had a distant, faraway look; he seemed to be looking at something I couldn't see, and he refused hand feeding.

Suddenly I suspected that Orville knew he was dying. Eating was no longer of paramount importance in his life; he was letting himself go.

Damn, damn, damn, I thought.

All day long I hovered around his cage, checking on him. At first he seemed to hold his own. But by the end of the day, he was failing fast.

As Karen prepared to leave after the hospital closed, she asked, "Shall I put your home number on for emergencies?"

"No," I murmured. "I'll take care of the recorder. I'm going to stay for a while." My eyes avoided Karen's as I added in a white lie, "I've got lots of charts to fill out. You go ahead. See you in the morning."

After Karen's departure, I turned my attention to Orville. Yes, the end was near. Orville was not destined to be the beneficiary of a medical miracle. No more effortless soaring and sailing above the mighty Lake Superior for Orville—at least, not in this body. I pulled up a chair and sat by his cage, not wanting to leave him alone.

Orville died early that hot August night.

4

Mrs. Mosely

Most injured wild creatures are dropped off and left with me. Occasionally an individual may stay around for the initial exam. It was not unusual for some to request a report of the outcome of a case. But once in a while, someone demanded more. Coping with these people was a task in itself.

"There's a woman up front with an owl," Karen announced to me as I performed surgery on a dog. "She hit it with her car. She says it's badly hurt. She wants you to look at it at once. I told her you were in surgery, but she insists on waiting."

I glanced at Karen; she wasn't kidding. "Tell her it'll be another fifteen minutes. Have her fill out an information sheet for the record. You know, species of owl, where it was hit—the usual stuff." Karen left, and I went back to work. Five minutes passed.

Karen popped in again, a slight smile on her face. "You're going to love this woman, Dr. Foster. Her name is Mrs. Mosely. She's neat. She has to be at least eighty years old, but her mind's as sharp as a tack. She's frantic about that owl, though. Can't you hurry?"

"Put her in the first exam room. Tell her I'll be only a few more minutes. You can turn off the anesthetic while you're here. I just have to close, and I'll be done."

Karen turned off the anesthetic and hurried away, as if on a higher mission in life.

I finished the surgery, made the dog comfortable and hurried off to find Mrs. Mosely almost in tears. While I was concerned for the owl, I couldn't help being fascinated by this woman.

Mrs. Mosely had white hair, fluffy with curls. Her sharp blue eyes sparkled behind her spectacles; she was very old, and she had an air about her that demanded attention. She wore a powder blue T-shirt with the word "Grandmother" stamped across the front, Madras shorts, and dashing blue sneakers. I liked her on sight.

"What's the problem?" I said softly, hoping her tears might abate.

"Oh, Dr. Foster, I feel so bad," she sobbed. "I've been driving for over fifty years, and this is the first animal I've hit." She swallowed, reined in her emotions and in a more even tone said, "You gotta save him!"

I gathered this was a command, so I set right to work. Inside a box on the table was a barred owl—on its back and seemingly stone-cold dead. I cringed, but said it anyway: "It may be too late. This bird may not be alive."

Fresh sobs racked Mrs. Mosely's small but very fit body. "Save him," she cried.

I promised to do my best. I picked up the bird with one hand and placed it on the table. As I felt the chest, I was amazed to feel a faint rapid pulse. I didn't quite believe it. I touched one

Barred owls are one of the most common owls of northern Wisconsin. After leaving the nest, baby owls spend three or four days learning to fly. During that period they perch on the ground or on stumps under their mother's watchful eye. This little fellow had been attacked by a stray dog. When healed, it was returned to its nest where the mother was still waiting.

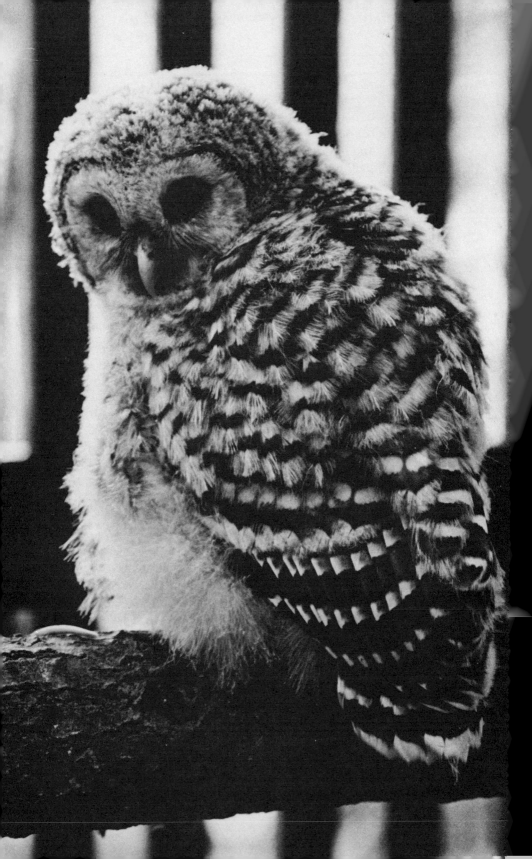

of the owl's large hazel blue eyes to check the corneal reflex. The eyelid closed slowly. "The owl is alive," I said, as if I had willed it. And now the bad news, I thought. "But it's comatose. It doesn't look good. But I'll try my best to save him." Then I backed off again, my fabricated optimism waning. "You never know, though."

Mrs. Mosely took off her glasses and wiped her sharp blue eyes. "I'm sorry to act this way. But it's all my fault. The poor bird!" She donned her spectacles and touched the owl, admiring its gray-brown feathers and the unique streaking on its belly. "He's so beautiful." She sighed. "Oh, I do so hope you can save him."

The obvious pleasure with which she appreciated the owl did me in. "Tell you what. If you leave your telephone number with the receptionist, I'll call you later today and let you know how he's doing." I picked up the owl as a cue for her to leave. I had two more surgeries before the afternoon appointments.

Mrs. Mosely began to move toward the exit. She was re-markably spry for her years, and I must admit I admired her snappy shorts and sneakers. A grin tugged at the corners of my mouth, but I managed to keep my face straight. Now Mrs. Mosely stood by the door. "I'll wait for your call," she said. The sharp blue eyes caught my eyes and held. "I figure it's okay to visit the owl when he gets better. Right?"

I hesitated. I didn't like to encourage visits to wild crea-tures. Human contact didn't benefit the patients, especially those who might return to the wild. Also visitors who dropped by and wandered around the hospital disrupted our routine. But in Mrs. Mosely's case, I relented, saying "Sure. Stop by anytime." I felt safe from Mrs. Mosely, since I didn't figure the owl to live long.

With a wave of the hand and a determined nod, Mrs. Mosely bid me farewell and wished me good luck with the owl.

I was going to need all the luck I could get. I dug up a textbook I thought might help. Since there was nothing on treating concussions or contusions in barred owls in any of my other books, I looked to a book on caged-bird medicine.

I turned to the parrot section, looking for dosages of drugs. A parrot and a barred owl weighed about the same; medication dosages should be similar, I concluded. So I started the owl on antibiotics and dexamethasone, an antiinflammatory steroid used to decrease swelling of the brain. Then I placed the owl in a dark cage, hoping for the best and returning to my routine of surgeries.

Except for the injections I'd given the owl, I was helpless. I could do nothing but wait for the outcome.

By late afternoon the owl's condition hadn't improved, but it hadn't grown worse, either. Just to be sure I hadn't missed anything, I radiographed the owl. Nothing new—no fracture or dislocations. I returned the owl to its cage and forced myself to telephone Mrs. Mosely.

"Mrs. Mosely," I said guardedly, "the owl's condition hasn't improved. But it's no worse. You can take heart in that." Then I retrenched. "Ah, still, I feel the prognosis is poor. Please do bear that in mind."

Mrs. Mosely wouldn't have any of that. "Well, it's good to know it's no worse. It'll probably be better in the morning."

Inwardly I groaned as I hung up. I wasn't as certain as Mrs. Mosely about the owl's future.

Before going home that night, I repeated the earlier injections on the owl. Having done my best, I said to the owl, "Get better for Mrs. Mosely," switched off the lights and wondered if the owl would be among the living in the morning.

Much to my surprise—it was!

The owl wasn't a whole lot better, but it was somewhat improved. He couldn't stand, but he did blink his big eyes at me, and his feet moved. Hallelujah! I thought; maybe the cause wasn't lost.

Promptly at nine o'clock, Mrs. Mosely telephoned. "The owl's better," I told her with some elation.

"I'll see you in about an hour," Mrs. Mosely replied.

"But, Mrs. Mosely, there's nothing you can do."

"Dr. Foster, you said I could visit him. I'll be right over." Click went the other end of the line. Mrs. Mosely was not to be deterred.

Forty-five minutes later, Mrs. Mosely charged through the front door of the hospital. "I'm here to see Stanfield," she announced to Karen.

Karen backed off. "Who's Stanfield?"

"Honey, that's what I've named the owl. Stanfield. Doesn't it have a marvelous ring to it? You just have to say it a few times to know it's right for him." She produced a paper sack from a tote bag that matched her shocking pink Bermuda shorts. "Here's some fresh doughnuts for you and Dr. Foster for doing such a good job on Stanfield."

Since the waiting room was full of barking dogs and hissing cats, Karen escorted Mrs. Mosely to the treatment room where the illustrious Stanfield was being housed. Mrs. Mosely pulled a chair up next to Stanfield's cage, sat down, and proceeded to eat all the doughnuts she had brought for Karen and me. In between doughnuts, she acted as a one-woman cheering section for Stanfield, urging him on, encouraging him to get well, telling him she was with him all the way. Oddly, Stanfield seemed to take in every word; his eyes never left her!

For the next four days I force-fed Stanfield by passing a stomach tube down the esophagus and giving him beef bouillon fortified with dextrose, vitamins, and minerals. Each day, Stanfield's guardian, Mrs. Mosely, visited him with doughnuts, words of encouragement, and bold strokes of loving affection on Stanfield's head.

By the end of the week, miracle of miracles, Stanfield could stand on a log and eat on his own. Though he was weak, he was improving.

On the eighth day, Mrs. Mosely announced, "I think Stanfield's going to be okay. Right?"

"Sure looks that way," I had to admit.

"Well, I want to be here when you release him. It'll make me feel good to see him fly off into the wild blue yonder. You know, as if I had a hand in curing him. Hope you don't mind?"

I nodded, obviously in over my head. "But," I said, "you must realize, it's not going to happen right away. Stanfield has to go through a couple of weeks of exercising to build up his muscles again. My brother Race is coming tomorrow to help me for the summer. He's good at getting birds in shape again."

Mrs. Mosely was pleased. She seemed to believe that I was flying in a world-renowned specialist just for Stanfield. She hauled off and gave me a big hug!

Now I looked forward to Race's arrival, not that I didn't under other circumstances. But Race was a veterinary student from my alma mater, Michigan State University, and he was very adept with wildlife. Not only did he have a sincere interest in wild creatures, but he had also received more formal training in avian physiology than I had. This was an invaluable asset in diagnosing and treating injured birds. Furthermore, he had a great sense of humor; work was more fun with Race around.

The day Race arrived, I told him about Stanfield and Mrs. Mosely. Race said, "Onward to the chore," and took Stanfield out of his cage to begin rehabilitative therapy.

This strengthening program consisted of two stages. The first several days involved nothing more than taking the bird outside, holding its feet, and moving the owl up and down. This motion prompted the involuntary extension of the wings, which assisted in eliminating the stiffness that had resulted from lack of use. The second stage was a more active regimen—tying a jess, a leashlike device, to one foot, then letting the bird fly a short circle overhead. This procedure progressed from a few minutes once a day to several fifteen- to twenty-minute sessions several times daily, until the bird was ready to fly on its own. In Stanfield's case, I surmised the exercises might take only ten to fourteen days; he had been flightless for a relatively short time.

The first two days of exercise for Stanfield went as planned. Meanwhile, Race was hitting it off outrageously with Mrs. Mosely. Now she brought Race fresh doughnuts, too, while saying to him, "Young man, I like your style." Of course Race joked and kidded with her, and Mrs. Mosely bloomed under Race's dark good looks and winning ways. She seemed to have an endless array of nifty sporting ensembles in bright colors. I had not imagined there were so many different colors in sneakers. Then things went slightly awry.

I was in the treatment room suturing a laceration on a small beagle. Race came in after the third day's exercise session with Stanfield, and his face was pale and somber, his eyes darting nervously around the room, as if he might be at a loss for words.

"What's the matter?" I demanded.

"It's Stanfield," he muttered.

"Stanfield? What about him? Isn't he doing well?" I bent over the anesthetized beagle to place the final stitch in his leg.

"That's not the problem. He's doing too well."

"Too well?" I glanced up at him. That hardly seemed likely. "What do you mean?"

Race groaned and muttered, "Stanfield slipped out of my hand somehow, and flew away."

"Oh, my God, what are we going to tell Mrs. Mosely?"

"I don't know," Race said. "She'll be crushed. Broken-hearted. Her specialist has let her down."

"She even postponed a trip to California so she could be here to see Stanfield off."

"Don't tell me. I know." My brother began to pace the room. "Maybe it's time to push the panic button."

"Well, at least we don't have to face her again today."

"Yeah, she was here before I lost Stanfield."

"Let's just wait until tomorrow when she comes in," I suggested. "You can tell her then."

Race whirled on me. "*You* tell her. You're the big-time doctor. I'm just a know-nothing student."

I grinned. "Ah, but you're the exercise specialist. You're the one who—"

"Don't tell me," Race said again. "I know, I know. I lost him!"

Promptly at ten o'clock the next morning, Mrs. Mosely waltzed through the hospital's front door, a bag of fresh doughnuts under each arm. Fortunately I was in the radiology room with an owner and his canine companion. As was her way, Mrs. Mosely, finding everyone occupied, marched directly to the treatment room to see Stanfield. Since the radiology room is right next door, I expected to hear an outburst almost immediately. But nothing happened. I listened more intently, and what did I hear? I heard Mrs. Mosely talking to Stanfield.

To say that I was shocked is putting it mildly. I excused myself and stepped into the treatment room to investigate.

Mrs. Mosely was peering into a cage that contained another barred owl, which Race had admitted earlier that morning. Evidently Mrs. Mosely had mistaken this owl for Stanfield. Bless us all, I thought, and quickly grabbed the record from the wall file behind her.

The chart indicated that this owl had been hit by a car, too. Race had diagnosed a small hairline fracture of the right femur, but the owl used its injured leg rather well. Without careful observation by an expert, this might have been Stanfield!

"Ah," said Mrs. Mosely turning to my presence, "I see you're on duty, Dr. Foster."

I cleared my throat and examined the chart carefully. "Yes, oh, yes, Mrs. Mosely."

"And do you expect to release Stanfield as Race told me, perhaps next week?"

I didn't have long to wrestle with my unwillingness to tell her the truth.

Race bolted into the room from around the corner where he'd been lurking, eavesdropping on the conversation. "Hi, Mrs. Mosely!" He beamed. "Great to see you."

"It's keen to see you, too," said Mrs. Mosely. "What about Stanfield?"

"Oh, yes, Stanfield." Race stood tall in the saddle now. "Stanfield is doing just super. But this morning I noticed, while exercising him, that he's going to need more therapy than I thought." He pointed to Stanfield with what I thought was an overly dramatic gesture. "See? Right there. Look closely at those wing muscles. We have to build those up much more. You wouldn't want him released with weak muscles, would you? It's going to be another three weeks or so."

Mrs. Mosely studied the bogus Stanfield intently. It was, of course, impossible to see the muscles under the feathers. Anyway, this owl's muscles were normal. But Mrs. Mosely fell victim to Race's charms. "I see what you mean. I'm glad you recognized that, Race. You're sharp. No doubt about it. You'd better keep him longer. I want the best for Stanfield."

With that, Mrs. Mosely handed Race his bag of fresh doughnuts. Calmly Race opened the bag, removed a doughnut, and began to eat it with relish. "Nothing like Mrs. Mosely's fresh doughnuts," he said. Despite the previous night's end-of-the-term celebration, his bloodshot eyes gleamed happily.

Three weeks later, Race and Mrs. Mosely released Stanfield II on schedule. It was a momentous occasion.

With tears in her bright blue eyes, Mrs. Mosely watched as Stanfield took to the sky. When the owl disappeared from view, she turned to Race, grabbed him, and kissed him lovingly on the cheek. "Thank you, Race," she said. "You did a fantastic job, and I'll never forget you." She hugged him tight. Then she paused before her departure and added, "I'll tell everyone what a wonderful doctor you are!"

Race replied smoothly, "Why, thank you, Mrs. Mosely."

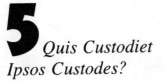

5 *Quis Custodiet*
Ipsos Custodes?

The challenge of treating and rehabilitating injured wildlife during that first year was formidable. In addition to many barred owls and seagulls, I worked on approximately seventy other patients representing twenty-three species, including belted kingfishers, four different species of hawks, and even a bald eagle.

Success in every case depended on appropriate medication and often delicate surgery plus a certain amount of sheer luck. Then, in the spring of 1979, an event happened where the ultimate outcome of a particular case was beyond my control. The wildlife practice involved more than the strict application of veterinary skills to injured wild patients.

The Department of Natural Resources (DNR) of Wisconsin is an enormous and powerful state governmental body. Its function is to oversee and regulate virtually every endeavor remotely related to national resources.

The DNR is departmentalized into various agencies and bureaus, each of which is expected to cope efficiently with a particular environmental responsibility. Some personnel are concerned only with air quality, for example, while other agencies reign over forestry and mining practices. Of course, there's a division whose territory is wildlife.

My differences with the DNR's wildlife office began early in my campaign to treat and release injured wildlife, and the conflict continues unabated. While I'd had a number of confrontations with DNR employees over the years, my first skirmish of real significance involved Little Joe, an orphaned otter.

During this period, I was practicing small-animal veterinary medicine at my hospital in Minocqua, while covering an-

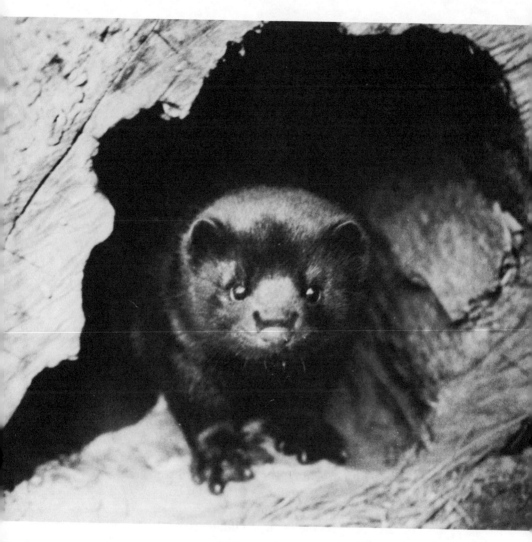

The mink, a cousin of the otter, is also a common north woods resident. This mink's mother was killed by a truck, and he was raised at the center and released.

other nearby clinic occasionally. Dr. T. J. Dunn and I had opened the Eagle River Animal Hospital, twenty-three miles east of Minocqua, in August 1978.

Since it was common knowledge throughout the north woods that I treated injured wildlife, the Eagle River Animal Hospital became a drop-off point for wild creatures in need of assistance, too. It was here on May 14, 1979, that the tiny motherless otter we named Little Joe first appeared.

A husky man entered and stepped up to the reception counter at the Eagle River Animal Hospital to be met by the enthusiastic and vivacious receptionist, Peggy.

"I'm the chief engineer for the new bridge on the county line road over Forest River," he said. "My name's Harold McDowny."

"What can I do for you?" asked Peggy, always eager to oblige.

"I have a baby otter in my car that needs help. One of the guys on the crew said he heard you take in wildlife and release 'em back into the wild. Is that true?"

Peggy, her personality suited to her job and a definite asset to the clinic, said eagerly, "That's right." Though we didn't get a great many wildlife patients in Eagle River, Peggy did most of the time-consuming work of nursing the injured wildlings back to health. She had endless patience and enjoyed every minute of her job. She was my chargé d'affaires when I was in Minocqua, and she took her work to heart. Peggy was quick to explain our policy about orphaned wildlife. "Dr. Dunn and Dr. Foster won't take the otter unless you're absolutely sure it's an orphan. They don't want any baby animals removed from their natural environment by mistake. Are you *sure* the baby otter is an orphan?"

"Positive," said McDowny. "We were digging by the river to put in some footings, and the bulldozer accidentally dug up the den. The adult darted out and was killed by one of our trucks on the road, I'm sorry to say. I checked her myself to be sure it wasn't a male. It was the mother all right. Her glands were full of milk. We dug out the nest and found just this one baby. No one knew what else to do, so I brought it here.''

"Bring the otter on in," said Peggy. "We'll take care of it.''

The engineer went out to his car and returned with the newborn otter wrapped in a red hooded sweat shirt with ''University of Wisconsin'' emblazoned on the front. "Here you go, miss. I sure hope you can help the little thing. You can keep the sweat shirt." He grinned. "I went to Notre Dame myself.''

Peggy accepted the bundle, and McDowny departed. She found Dr. Dunn in the radiology room, examining a set of X-rays. Said Peggy triumphantly, "We have a new patient. A baby otter!'' Carefully she unfolded the sweat shirt for Dr. Dunn, and together they examined the helpless five-inch-long creature.

Dr. Dunn palpated the otter all over to be sure there were no injuries. The little creature's short but stout legs flailed harmlessly, indicating to Dr. Dunn that the tiny otter was in fine shape.

I had spent my first year out of veterinary school working with Dr. Dunn in Rhinelander. Never did I cease to be impressed with his ability to feel things in his patients. He could detect minor abnormalities in a dog's or cat's abdomen—abnormalities that other veterinarians might have missed. He had magic fingers, no doubt about it. Meanwhile, he was probably the finest veterinary diagnostician I'd seen, including those at universities. I felt fortunate to have had the opportunity to train with him before venturing out on my own in Minocqua; and I had jumped at the chance to start the clinic in Eagle River with him a couple of years later.

Now he looked up at Peggy and said, "This little fellow is going to mean an awful lot of work for us, Peggy.''

Peggy didn't mind. "I can't get over how helpless he is. Look. His eyes aren't even open yet. He's the cutest little thing I ever saw.''

Dr. Dunn grinned at Peggy, saying, "Yes, he's adorable. But at this age a small mammal should be fed every two hours or so. I'm going over to Minocqua tonight. I can take him to Rory and Linda, if you like.''

''Oh, no,'' Peggy was quick to respond. ''I can take care of him. I've got time, and I know how to do it. I raised three orphaned squirrels last year. Remember? I'll do everything exactly the way you tell me. Can I call Dr. Foster to see if it's okay with him?''

''Why not?'' said Dr. Dunn. ''He'll be glad to hear you're ready, willing, and able.''

When Peggy telephoned, I couldn't do anything but agree. Linda and I had an orphaned owl, two fawns, two baby robins, and our one-year-old daughter Ali. Our cup runneth over! Anyway, Peggy was dedicated and capable. If things didn't go well for the otter, it wouldn't be Peggy's fault.

Following Dr. Dunn's instructions, Peggy started Little Joe on Esbilac, a commercial milk replacement for animals, which contains all the necessary nutrients for proper growth. Additionally, she put the tiny otter to bed on a heating pad night and day to prevent hypothermia.

Educated to the acceptable routine, Peggy took complete charge of Little Joe's case. She fed him with an eyedropper every two hours from 6:00 A.M. until 10:00 P.M. She awakened at 2:00 A.M. to ensure that Little Joe's appetite was satisfied.

In two weeks, it was obvious to one and all that Little Joe was healthy and growing. We began to plan ahead for his return to the wild. As soon as we weaned him, we would transfer him to an outdoor location and gradually reduce the amount of human contact. With the aid of a small pool we felt we could teach him to catch fish, a skill that would be vital to his survival in the wild. The task wouldn't be easy, but we had accomplished similar feats with other mammals. We felt Little Joe had a good chance of living a long and successful life. Eventually, of course, we expected to release him in the wilds of northern Wisconsin far from human inhabitants. Unfortunately, we never had the opportunity to carry out our plans.

A frantic Peggy telephoned me at eight o'clock on a June morning with the devastating news. "Dr. Foster, you've got to do something!"

I sensed Peggy was near tears. "What is it, Peggy?"

"A DNR worker just came and took Little Joe," she cried.

"Start from the beginning. Try to get hold of yourself. What happened?"

Peggy pulled herself together and managed, "I got to work at seven-thirty as usual. This DNR warden just walked in unannounced and took him. Dr. Dunn wasn't here yet. I didn't want to give up Little Joe. But the warden said I had to."

"Did he say anything else?"

"He said he'd heard we had a baby otter here. Then he told me they needed one to sell. He mentioned a place called Wild Animal Haven."

"What's Wild Animal Haven?" I'd never heard of it.

But Peggy knew. "It's a filthy tourist attraction about ten miles south of town. They sell gifts and keep some wild animals in pens. I was down there once. It was so dirty and disgusting I never went again. I even called the humane officer, but he couldn't do anything about it."

Peggy didn't need to say more. I knew the type of place she described. The state of Wisconsin is littered with so-called wildlife exhibits, or roadside zoos. Unlike true zoological gardens, the roadside zoos are run mostly by amateurs with purely economic motives. A properly run zoo, in addition to providing a good environment for wildlife, is an educational institution and very often offers opportunities for breeding rare and endangered species. A genuine concern for the individual animal and species and a dedication to learning are the qualities that distinguish the true zoo from a roadside menagerie.

Another important difference lies in the care provided to the animals. The crowding that all too often marks the roadside zoos inevitably leads to poor physical and mental health for the animals and can manifest itself in bizarre behavior and unnatural conflicts. Sanitation is another major problem. In roadside wildlife exhibits, cages and pens tend to be improperly cleaned which leads to disease and parasitism.

I was convinced, as a result of my conversation with Peggy, that Wild Animal Haven was a typical roadside exhibit that purchased wild animals and displayed them for entertainment or amusement only. Furious, I picked up the telephone and called the DNR area field office.

"This is Dr. Rory Foster, veterinarian," I said. "I'm calling about an incident that occurred about an hour ago at the Eagle River Animal Hospital."

"Hold on, please," said the cool voice.

Five minutes later, a peevish voice said, "This is Jack Einer. Can I help you, Mr. Foster?"

"Yes," I snapped. "Are you aware of the otter that was confiscated from my hospital this morning by one of your wardens?"

"I know of it."

"I'm calling to file a complaint. That otter was brought to us as an orphan. We intended to release him back into the wild. We didn't raise him to be sold."

"Mr. Foster, all wildlife belongs to the DNR, according to state statute. We can do what we want with them."

"Does that include walking into a veterinary hospital without notice and taking patients to sell to half-assed tourist traps like Wild Animal Haven?" I was really rolling; there's simply no way to describe how angry I was. I raged on: "Are you aware that Wild Animal Haven is filthy and lacks proper facilities for animals? That otter was a patient under veterinary care. You can't just walk in and take a patient. For God's sake, no one even called to see if the otter was healthy!"

"That's for us to decide, Mr. Foster. It's none of your concern. According to state statute—"

I pulled the telephone away from my ear so that I wouldn't have to listen to him recite the state statute to me. Finally, I heard his voice winding down, and I cut in, saying, "How much did you get paid for the otter?"

"Three hundred dollars," said Jack Einer icily. "You can check the DNR general fund accounting, if you feel the need."

With that, I lost all control. "Mr. Einer, you're a bastard!"

"What was that, Mr. Foster?"

"You're a bastard!" I shouted.

The telephone clicked in my ear. Jack Einer had hung up.

Next I telephoned the regional office of the DNR. The result was the same—callous indifference toward the life of an otter. All I heard was more about laws, regulations, and statutes. Nobody gave a damn about Little Joe and his future.

Little Joe remained at Wild Animal Haven for two months—until he died. The veterinarian who saw him shortly before his death told me that Little Joe died of distemper, a preventable disease if proper immunization procedures have been followed.

Fourteen months later, after numerous complaints about the degrading conditions of Wild Animal Haven, public pressure caused the place to be closed down. But it was too late for Little Joe.

After my angry outburst, the area DNR personnel never again sold a patient from one of my hospitals. But I couldn't help wondering about other orphaned wildlings who didn't come to us, especially those in other parts of the state. How many other Little Joes had been sold to similar outlets?

It was a sad day when the Department of Natural Resources, a public agency created to be the guardian of wildlife, could participate in such activities. It brought to my mind an old Latin phrase: *Quid custodiet ipsos custodes?* Who shall guard the guardians?

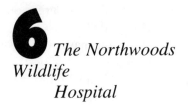

6 The Northwoods Wildlife Hospital

One evening, after an exhausting day at the clinic, I came home and announced to Linda, "We're going to have to do something. I've got seventeen cages at the hospital—all intended for dogs and cats. Today fourteen of those cages were occupied by wildlife." I sank down wearily in a chair in the living room. "That doesn't include the fawn here at home or the three owls in the basement; and tomorrow I'm supposed to get a blue jay with a broken wing and a pileated woodpecker that had the top half of his beak shot off." I looked up at Linda, who was standing by, and added, "Can you imagine anyone shooting at a pileated woodpecker?"

Linda shook her head in dismay. "No, I can't. But I can't imagine anyone shooting a bald eagle, either. Last year," she reminded me, "there were two shot around here, not to mention the loon you had last month with six shotgun pellets in it!"

I rubbed my face, hoping the memory would go away. But it didn't. One of the owls in our basement had been shot, too. But now I had reached an impasse. There was no more room at the inn. I heard myself say angrily, "What am I going to do? I had to send a dog home today too soon after knee surgery. That's not right. He should've stayed in the hospital."

Linda settled on the sofa across the room. "Can't you send some of the wildlife to someone else?"

"To whom?" I asked almost bitterly. The nearest treatment center was in St. Paul, Minnesota, at the university. They only took in birds of prey, and they were a good 180 miles from us. Most people simply couldn't take the time to make the trip.

Linda and I sat in silence for a while, pondering our dilemma. Finally, she said, "What can we do?"

I glanced up at her hopefully. "I did have a brainstorm today."

In Linda I had the perfect audience for my brainstorm, and suddenly the situation didn't seem so bleak. "Let's have a Crown Royal."

Linda went to the kitchen and returned with a couple of drinks. Once I was settled securely in my easy chair with a drink in my hand and she had moved back to the sofa, I took a sip of my drink and looked into the far distance. "Well, I was thinking. Just thinking, mind you. But why not start a nonprofit organization to care for injured wildlife?"

"That's a good idea!"

My eyes swung back to her. "You mean it?"

"Yes, it's a super-good idea."

"We could raise funds and solicit members," I told her, leaning forward in anticipation. "Like the Sierra Club or the Audubon Society. Eventually we could build a real wildlife hospital. We could donate the land and connect it with a hallway to the existing animal hospital. Then we wouldn't have to duplicate the expensive hospital equipment. Surgery and X-rays could still be done on the clinic side of the building, while the hospitalization and rehabilitation would be done at the wildlife center."

Linda's blue eyes widened with excitement. "Fantastic! Why didn't we think of this before?"

Satisfied that I had a willing partner, I took a sip of my drink and said, "I guess we never realized how busy we'd get treating wildlife!"

"I can see it now," said Linda. "In a wildlife hospital, the patients could have better care."

"And we could even develop a wildlife education program geared toward preventing the abuse we keep seeing!"

Linda and I stayed up until 2:30 A.M., hashing it all out,

imagining the unique possibilities that the Northwoods Wildlife Hospital and Rehabilitation Center could offer. It was, to our way of thinking, a triumphant proposal.

The next morning, over breakfast, the idea appeared absolutely sterling in our mind's eye. We would do it; and it all seemed so right.

At the office that day, I admitted the blue jay and the pileated woodpecker. Now I was down to one vacant cage. If my idea had been sterling, now it was absolutely crucial. I had no other choice. It was either build on an addition or stop treating injured wildlife—not much of a choice. I knew what I wanted.

By late summer of 1979, the project was under way. Eleven interested community members, along with Linda and me, had applied for and received nonprofit tax-exempt status for the Northwoods Wildlife Hospital and Rehabilitation Center. Our membership drive had culminated in three hundred eager supporters. We began a building fund for the eventual construction of the wildlife hospital. But to our astonishment, opposition began to surface.

To this day I have difficulty understanding the motives of those who sought to destroy our project. No public funds were solicited, and those from the private sector were given voluntarily. Further, no monies were allocated to any director or to me. I gave my time freely and donated all medical and surgical supplies. But many individuals were publicly opposed to our program; they represented diverse sectors of the population, and they opposed us most vocally.

Letters appeared in our area newspaper, *The Lakeland Times*, taking a stand against the Northwoods Wildlife Hospital and Rehabilitation Center (NWHRC). Reasons for being against the project varied widely, but one theme surfaced again and again: the belief that our efforts would do little to aid wild populations.

Time after time I pointed out publicly that our aim was not to assist wild populations. The directors of our group realized that saving one wild creature was not important to the wild population as a whole, except when dealing with endangered species. This saving grace, though, was singularly crucial to the individual, and here was our motive. Our work was humanitarian, not ecological. It was also practical; if a person injured a wildling, there was no place else to take the bird or animal for treatment. All too often, in areas without interested veterinarians or a project like NWHRC, injured wildlife ended up being mistreated, or worse yet, being kept as pets. Our project promised to end that situation in our area, if nothing else.

It was slow going, but eventually the critics of the NWHRC gained momentum. They threatened our credibility and our very existence.

Two of the more outspoken critics were well known and were liked by longtime area residents. One of them owned a wildlife art gallery and gift shop; the other owned a roadside zoo in the state. Their damaging statements found their way into a statewide newspaper, *The Milwaukee Sentinel,* where they blasted the NWHRC.

By September, I decided my only hope was to try to arrange some kind of truce with these determined people. I ventured forth resolutely to the roadside wildlife exhibit to meet the owner.

The owner was busy when I arrived at his establishment. While I waited, I strolled around the wildlife display to see the animals. Except for the deer and some scattered goats, pigs, and ducks running loose, most of the wildlife was confined to small rectangular or circular cages arranged in rows among dirt paths from which the paying public could view the wildlife.

My first stop was at an otter cage; it contained two oblong pools of water, each about ten feet in diameter. Four otters frolicked in the blue water, wrestling, tugging, playfully biting one another. I stood before the cage, smiling at the antics of the otters. Then a red-haired woman and two adolescent boys came up to the cage.

Almost immediately the two boys began tossing caramel popcorn into the cage. The otters went for the treats. Soon a quarrel broke out between the two largest otters as they fought over the caramel popcorn.

The boys continued to toss popcorn into the cage, enjoying the havoc they were creating. Suddenly I couldn't stand it any longer. Still I kept a rein on my temper.

"Hey, guys," I said evenly. "I don't want to spoil your fun, but caramel popcorn isn't good for otters."

Startled by my words, the boys stopped their popcorn barrage and stared up at me blankly. Their mother joined them, giving me a glaring look. Silently they turned on their heels and headed up the path.

My next stop was at a cage that contained a fox. A small sign on the front of the cage read: Artic Fox. Someone didn't know how to spell. Surely this was an Arctic fox!

I moved on to pause before a cage housing two of our state mammals; two badgers paced back and forth nervously within a fifteen-foot-long enclosure. Their stout and powerful bodies went one way, only to turn abruptly and return in the direction from which they came. In the few minutes I stood before the cage, I counted this unending march from one end of the cage to the other. One badger repeated the trip twenty-seven times, while the other pursued a similar course on the opposite side of the pen, though its monotony was broken after every fifth or sixth pass with a side excursion to the cage wall, where it pressed its head against the wire, as if searching for an exit. These badgers were stir crazy, but the first one had long ago abandoned hope of escape. I felt the sting of tears in my eyes.

If the floor of the cage, like all others, had not been concrete, these badgers, using all four legs, could have dug a hole to freedom in less than a minute. Badgers are designed to dig, and their digging ability is unparalleled in the mammal world. They also adore digging; it is their nature, just as swimming is a delight to otters. But these two badgers were doomed to pacing. I moved on, shaking my head dismally.

Inside a circular cage about ten feet in diameter and sixteen feet high, a lone bobcat sat on a platform, nodding in sleep.

Despite my advance, the cat didn't move a muscle. His eyes opened only in slits. When I spoke to him softly and gently, he yawned in boredom.

As his mouth opened in a wide yawn, I checked his teeth. His large fangs, the canine teeth, were missing. No doubt they had been pulled out intentionally to prevent injury during handling, a common practice at roadside zoos. Meanwhile, below the bobcat's platform, a swarm of flies buzzed relentlessly around a recent pile of excrement. Hard for the cat to bury it in concrete, I thought wearily.

The more I saw, the less I liked what I saw. Here was mistreatment of the worst sort.

A majestic timber wolf lived alone in his cage. Like the bobcat, he was allowed a platform on which to sit and view the world, dull as his world was. A wild wolf's range in a natural state covers four hundred square miles. I judged the space in which the timber wolf lived to be no more than seventy-five square feet. I had seen more than enough to last me the rest of my life. God, how I hated these zoos.

I hurried along another path. Once again I encountered the red-haired woman with her two boys. They were feeding what appeared to be a bottle of orange soda through the bars of a cage to an adult black bear. Next to the bear's cage was a machine where they had purchased the bottle. The machine carried these words: Bear Soda—35¢!

Now I was walking more swiftly, more angrily toward the exit. Adjacent to the gate a red-tailed hawk sat on a post. Around his right leg a metal chain had been fastened to prevent escape. Abruptly I stopped and stared at him.

He stared back at me, his beady eyes seeming to tell me much.

His name was Ulysses, according to a sign on the post.

"Ulysses," I said, "I'll bet you'd like to fly away again."

Of course, he didn't answer. But during this brief interlude, yes, he told me much.

To see this healthy-looking, beautiful creature confined, kept on display for profit, tethered forever, was the final straw. This confirmed my belief in the inherent cruelty of roadside zoos. This one was relatively clean, but cleanliness just wasn't enough. The creatures trapped here knew they lived without hope of freedom. I knew it. And if others had stopped to think about it, they would have known it, too!

Then and there I concluded that our program didn't need the approval of this man who professed to love wildlife—yet owned a roadside zoo. A man like that would never be able to see the light of reason; and so, depressed by my visit, but more determined than ever, I took my departure.

In addition to opposition from private citizens such as the roadside zoo owner, we received criticism from employees of the Department of Natural Resources. Two area game wardens hampered our efforts; one of them wrote a letter to the local newspaper protesting our work.

His feelings toward injured wildlings was upsetting to those of us who were committed to saving wild creatures. He told me once that any fawn injured to the extent that its care would require over seventy-two hours in captivity should be "knocked in the head."

Another day, for no reason at all, this same public employee threatened to revoke my rehabilitative permit, which I had to have to legally treat injured wildlife in Wisconsin. And still another time, he said to me, "I expect to ticket anyone who brings you an injured creature on the grounds that, during its transport to the hospital, the person temporarily in possession will be technically in violation of the law."

In addition to the local DNR employees' opposition, I received substantial criticism from DNR policymakers in Madison, Wisconsin. Herbert Bodin, the DNR staff biologist, for instance, wrote me a letter complaining about our wildlife work. By treating individual birds and mammals, he said, I created a wrong impression of wildlife to the public. People should be concerned with populations, not with individual birds and animals, he claimed.

Having digested the letter, I placed a telephone call to Herbert Bodin. "This is Dr. Foster in Minocqua," I said. "I'm calling about your letter protesting our assistance to individual creatures."

"Yes, I wrote that letter," said Bodin.

"I have a question that I hope you can answer for me." I was fired up, and I hoped my voice didn't betray my ire. "Why is it illegal in Wisconsin to shoot *one* deer out of season or chase *one* loon with a motorboat?"

"Why is it illegal? I'll tell you why. Because we don't want people to do those things. That should be obvious, Dr. Foster."

"It is obvious to me, Mr. Bodin. But I wanted to hear *you* say it. That's all. Isn't it ironic that your laws do protect individuals? I should think that might give the public the wrong impression of wildlife. After all, individuals aren't important—remember? Not according to your letter!"

Though he didn't back off, I had made my point. I hoped he would think a bit more carefully before writing to me again spouting nonsense.

Perhaps the most damaging letter was written to *The Lakeland Times* by Ray Schoder, dean of the College of Natural Resources, University of Wisconsin, Stevens Point. Schoder attacked our program on the basis of several imaginative points.

He feared disease might spread from wildlife hospitals to wild populations. Further, he was against treating too many different species; the project might be more acceptable, at least to him, if we confined our treatment to birds of prey only or to endangered species.

The letter irritated me beyond words. The least he could have done was telephone me personally before attacking me in public. It struck me as very odd that a college dean from an outside area would write a letter at all.

Since I have always believed in confronting opponents, I

picked up the telephone and called Schoder directly. I told him who I was and then said, "I'd like to hear your theory of how disease spreads from a wildlife hospital to wild populations. Do you have any evidence that this is a real concern?" I was trying to keep an open mind, while controlling my temper. It wasn't easy. But so far, okay.

Schoder responded, "As a matter of fact, duck plague, a viral disease, has affected a great number of wild ducks in this country in a similar manner—"

"Wait a minute," I said. "If I recall my epidemiology correctly, duck plague was introduced to this country by a ship from Europe that carried domestic ducks. That had absolutely nothing to do with wildlife rehabilitation."

"Well, that's true, but—"

"Tell me, Mr. Schoder, do you know of one case of a wildlife rehabilitator being responsible for any disease in wildlife populations?"

"Well, no, not really . . ." Suddenly he was hedging.

"You mean," I said, hearing my voice rise, "that you wrote a public letter criticizing our project on that basis, and that such a case has never, to your knowledge, occurred?"

"Well . . ." Schoder began lamely.

Suddenly I felt much better. "While I have you on the phone, Schoder—you did say in your letter that you would graciously consent to our project if we confined our treatment to birds of prey or endangered species only, right? Well, suppose we follow your advice. Just suppose that. What will I do with the next loon I get with a fishhook in its wing? Turn it away because it's not a bird of prey and not endangered? Answer that one." I didn't wait for his answer, though. "Or what if we get a blue heron with a broken wing, and suppose I know I can fix that wing and release the heron? Why should you or anyone else care if I spend my time treating cases like those?" I paused for breath.

Schoder didn't answer.

I closed the conversation quick and slammed the phone into its cradle, still baffled, though considerably relieved, and pleased by my brave opponent's hasty retreat.

Three weeks later, however, I saw Schoder's position in another light. He had been appointed to the state governing board of the Department of Natural Resources.

Our opponents had no rational basis for their fierce opposition, but the bitter debate was costly to our organization. Many potential members refused to join for fear the project might cease to exist. The controversy sapped the morale and energy of some of the board members to such a point that several of them handed in their resignations. Unfortunately, the public debate spilled over into my private life, too.

One day Linda was grocery shopping when a man approached her. She'd never seen him before in her life, but he had this to say: "Tell your husband that there's a lot of us town folk that don't agree with what he's doing."

His tone of voice was so threatening that Linda left her grocery basket where it stood, fled to the car, and drove home crying.

At a local high school football game one evening, a dentist approached me and asked, "How can you justify spending money on wildlife when the school doesn't have enough money for new football equipment?"

To which I replied, "How can you justify playing golf?"

The golfer-dentist backed off and went his way.

The negative aspects of the bitter controversy spilled over into our finances as well. I applied for a loan from a local bank

The author (left) *and Dr. Marty Smith perform surgery to remove a fishhook buried deep in a loon's stomach. Each year the hospital treats many water birds, unwittingly injured by fishermen.*

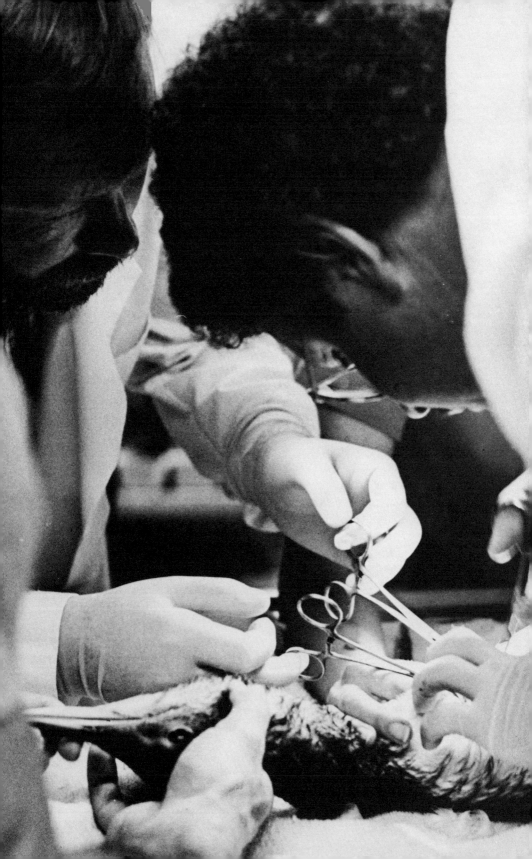

to build the wildlife hospital. I was one of the founders of the bank, and I served on the board of directors. Certainly I'd find friends here.

I was told that the loan would be denied unless other area banks participated. My ability to repay the loan was not in question; the Northwoods Wildlife Hospital was just too controversial for the bank to handle alone. They required additional backing, according to the loan officer. I later resigned as a member of the board of directors.

In the face of all this opposition, I continued to treat injured wildlife. Working with these patients each day helped me maintain my enthusiasm when the outlook was truly bleak. I needed all the encouragement I could get, and seeing a wild creature made well, seeing it turned free to live out its life in peace and harmony with nature was the best medicine for me.

In the fall, Karen, my assistant, asked me a question I'd been asked many times by others during these past months: "Dr. Foster, do you regret starting the whole wildlife thing? I mean, isn't it a kind of thorn in your side?"

I looked at Karen thoughtfully, but instead of answering her question, I said, "How about going with me to release that loon we've been taking care of?"

Karen was pleased to be included in the loon's release. So we departed the hospital, leaving Carrie, our part-time receptionist, in charge, and Karen and I drove out to Trout Lake to release the loon we had nursed back to health after a fishhook injury.

I stopped the car along the shoreline of Trout Lake, the largest body of water in the area, and we got out, carrying the box that contained Lunar. The moment I opened the box, the nine-pound loon sprang free and dived into the crystal-clear water of Trout Lake.

We stood there for a while, watching Lunar swim powerfully toward deep water. Then he was gone from sight. Shortly he surfaced several hundred yards away, his loud haunting cry shattering the stillness of the early afternoon. A thrill ran up my spine as I watched Lunar dive again. When he came up, he tested his wings. Using his legs he ran across the choppy water into the wind for nearly a quarter of a mile, the normal distance required for a loon to acquire the speed to become airborne. Now slowly he gained altitude and flew toward the narrows between North and South Trout Lake.

When Lunar was only a speck on the distant horizon, I turned to Karen.

"No need to say anything," she said. "I understand."

1 On the Wild Side

A number of other individuals were strongly in favor of the Northwoods Wildlife Hospital. Fortunately for us they spoke up, or all might have been lost.

Perhaps the most helpful commentator at the height of the controversy was Dr. Pat Redig, co-founder and chief veterinarian of the National Raptor (Bird of Prey) Center at the University of Minnesota. Dr. Redig appeared at a fund raiser and wrote to newspapers, discussing the Northwoods Wildlife Hospital in professional and philosophical terms, and this helped enormously.

He also tactfully avoided mentioning my minor—but very embarrassing—goofs. Dr. Redig didn't mention the thirty or forty times I'd called on him for badly needed advice, for example. And he failed to detail my periodic hawk identification problems—like the time I sent him a rare Cooper's hawk, which somehow managed to transform itself into a common broad-winged hawk on its way to the university. Most conveniently, he forgot to mention the time I fed the wrong chipmunk to a great horned owl!

The chipmunk had come into the hospital with a broken back. Since there was nothing I could do for it, I put it to sleep humanely with an injection. But somehow I got this animal mixed up with a chipmunk that had been accidentally hit and killed by a car that very same day.

Occasionally we fed road-killed small mammals to hospitalized birds of prey, and I inadvertently fed the wrong chipmunk to Alex, the recuperating great horned owl, prior to leaving work one evening.

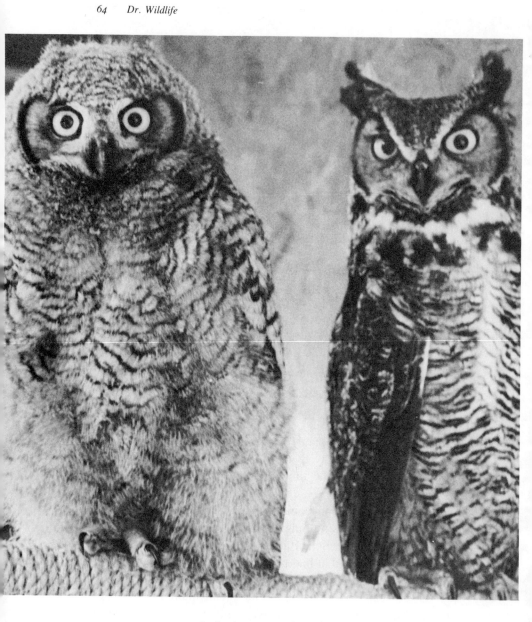

Left: *immature barred owl;*
Right: *mature great horned owl.*

The next morning, I discovered Alex, lying in the bottom of his cage, his feet pointing to the ceiling comatose. I was frantic. What had gone wrong?

I leafed through my books, but I couldn't find any disease of owls with Alex's clinical record. No disease struck so fast, so sure. Then it hit me: I had discovered a rare new disease!

A consultation was in order. I grabbed the telephone and placed a call to Dr. Redig.

Said Dr. Redig, "What did you feed Alex yesterday?"

"A chipmunk," I said . . . and then it dawned on me.

The next day the pentobarbitol from the chipmunk Alex had eaten wore off. Our great horned owl awoke from his deep sleep in good form. In fact, he had never felt better. I could tell; I was feeling just wonderful myself!

Dr. Redig's letter, printed in *The Lakeland Times,* was timely and helpful:

I have followed with considerable interest the building negative editorial comment surrounding the proposal of Dr. Rory Foster of the Northwoods Wildlife Hospital and Rehabilitation Center to develop a facility for medical care and research of, and public education toward, the wildlife of northern Wisconsin.

It is most important to realize that since its inception, Dr. Foster's proposal has been directed at integrating all three of the aforementioned facets, whereas critics have focused almost entirely on what they feel are the questionable aspects of the rehabilitation of injured wildlife alone.

My own facility has provided care for over 1,500 birds of prey since 1972, and of these 42 percent were released. Post-release monitoring of recovered eagles has documented the successful return of these birds to the wild and evidence of several rejoining the breeding population.

The clinical setting has provided extensive opportunities for developing special techniques in avian anesthesia, orthopedic surgery, and for documenting the effects of environmental toxins (pollutants) such as lead, pesticides, and strychnine as well as the opportunity for several veterinary and graduate students to learn material that can be directly applied to the management of wildlife.

Lastly, very positive presentation of our program to the public by the local news media has profoundly sensitized the people of the Twin Cities area to the plight of much of our wildlife, and has helped people to realize the very direct ways in which many of our accepted ways of living affect the environment and wildlife.

Our facilities are open to the public and we especially encourage young people to visit and see first-hand how the callous indifference of many people results in some very special and beautiful birds being shot, trapped, forcibly removed from their nests and fed inadequate diets, or dying in violent tremors from ingestion of toxic substances.

Such an experience has produced a firm resolve in the minds of the many thousands that have visited that their lives will be filled with a much deeper concern for other living creatures.

I have thoroughly reviewed Dr. Foster's proposal and conferred with him at length on the subject. His commitment to the research and public education aspects of wildlife medicine are as well developed as his concern for straightforward rehabilitation.

There is a genuine need for his interest and dedication, and it would be a real tribute to the understanding and concern that the people of northern Wisconsin have for their beautiful and unique wildlife resources to give their support to this project.

Sincerely,
Patrick T. Redig, D.V.M.
National Raptor. Research
and Rehabilitation Center
University of Minnesota

Encouraging and enlightening statements like Dr. Redig's brought a sense of rightness to my uphill battle. This sort of clear thinking assisted me in shouldering the burden I had lifted. In reading his letter, I knew my goal was feasible and reasonable. There was no turning back for me. This was not just a cause, but a way of life. Nothing could or would deter me. Well, at least I hoped not.

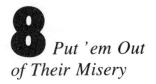

8 *Put 'em Out of Their Misery*

The public debate over the philosophy of treating and releasing injured wildlife subsided over the long winter months. At least for the moment the media had lost interest in the subject. But dealing with those who disagreed with our work on a personal level proved to be just as bitter and harsh.

On the night of June 12, 1980, I was awakened by the shrill ringing of the telephone. I reached out, pulled the phone into bed with me, and answered sleepily, "Dr. Foster speaking."

"This is Dick Simmons," the voice on the other end of the line said. "I just hit a fawn with my car. It's still alive. I read about you in the newspaper when I was up here last summer. Are you still treating wildlife?"

I came awake in a hurry now. "Sure. Where are you? I'll come right out."

"I'm calling from the Sportsman's Bar in Lake Tomahawk. I drove up here to make the call. The fawn is back by the junction of County D and Highway Forty-seven. I'll meet you there. I'll show you where the fawn is."

"No problem. I know where you mean. I'll be there in ten minutes."

"I had to report the accident to the police. I think they called the game warden. He might be there, too."

I thanked him for his call, promising to be right along.

I dressed quickly in the dark—it was 11:52 P.M. by the bedside clock—trying not to awaken Linda and Ali. The ring of the phone hadn't roused them, and I saw no need to disturb them. I hurried from the bedroom to encounter Tenille, our golden retriever. She greeted me with a friendly wag of her tail, and together we ran downstairs, through the dark basement, and into the garage. Tenille jumped into the Bronco beside me, and we were off.

"Hang on, Tenille," I cautioned her. "This is going to be a fast drive."

Tenille cocked her head at me, as if understanding perfectly.

Since the DNR had been notified about the injured fawn, I didn't know what was ahead of me. Once, the year before, the DNR men had beaten me to a car-struck fawn. They had shot it before I arrived.

I realized, of course, that in some cases humane euthanasia of an injured wild animal was necessary to prevent needless suffering, but I reserved this option for wildlings that had no chance of recovery, such as those with broken backs. Many wardens and other law-enforcement officials, however, opted for euthanasia immediately. Mostly they didn't bother to examine the injured creature at all. One warden had callously described the shooting of injured creatures as "lead poisoning"!

"Sit tight," I called out to Tenille. "We're almost there." I floored the Bronco as we left the gravel road and turned onto County D. Soon we pulled up to the intersection at Highway 47 behind a parked car, a blue Lincoln Continental with Illinois license plates. No doubt my caller was one of the many summer residents in our area.

I glanced around and spotted a man with a flashlight over near the ditch, not far from the car. "Stay, Tenille," I said, as I prepared to open the door to the Bronco. Just then a car pulled up from the other direction. Damn! It was probably the warden.

It was. He jumped from his car and headed for the ditch.

I followed, and we met at the ditch where the man stood holding the flashlight.

I hadn't met this warden before. He was in his early twenties, muscular in build. His pleasant face and blond hair reminded me of a lifeguard rather than a warden. Must be a summer trainee, I decided.

The man from Illinois was twice the age of the warden. He was strongly built and distinguished in appearance. Considering the circumstances, he was remarkably calm. Most motorists who had struck a deer were shaken and agitated. Not this man.

"I'm Dick Simmons," he said, extending his hand to the uniformed DNR man. "You must be the warden." They shook hands. Then he turned to me.

"I'm Rory Foster. It's good to meet you. I wish we could meet under different circumstances, though. Where's the fawn?"

He pointed the flashlight at a clump of grass a few feet away. Lying there was a spotted fawn.

The warden returned to his car to retrieve his clipboard. Now the questioning of Mr. Simmons began.

I turned on my flashlight and began to examine the fawn. A three-inch laceration above the eye caught my attention immediately. The wound had bled profusely. The entire right half of the fawn's face was bright red with blood.

While the warden questioned Simmons, I continued checking the fawn. I ran my hands over all four of its legs. No fracture was detectable. Next I felt along the dorsal processes of the vertebra. All were in line and evenly spaced. Good, I thought with satisfaction; no spinal cord damage.

The color of the conjunctiva—the tissue under the eye— was a normal pink; here was a good indication of acceptable blood pressure, which indicated no internal bleeding.

I had a gut feeling that the fawn had been hit on the head only. She was more than likely suffering from nothing more than the obvious laceration that had knocked her out. I was elated. There was hope.

The warden finished questioning Simmons and turned to the fawn. He was ten feet away, and his glance was brief. "May as well put it out of its misery. Look at all that blood. I'll get my pistol from the car."

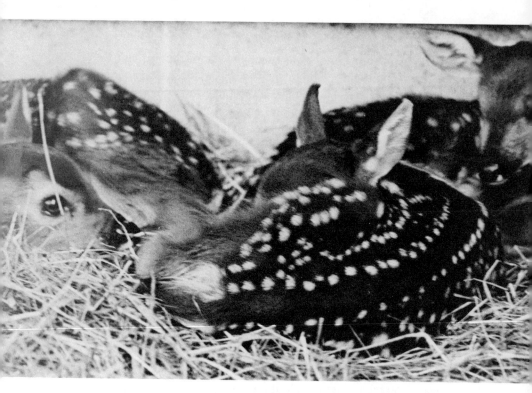

*Three fawns whose mothers were killed by cars.
In the spring and early summer the death of a doe
usually means that her fawn will starve unless it
is rescued and hand-raised.*

I wanted to avoid an angry confrontation, but with my heartbeat pounding double time in my chest, I doubted my ability to control myself. "Wait a minute," I said sharply. "I've examined the fawn. She may not be badly injured."

He paused in his pursuit of the pistol. "What do you mean? Look at it. It's just laying there suffering. Shooting it is the only humane thing to do."

"That fawn's unconscious. How could she be suffering? She can't feel anything!"

The warden glared at me. His eyes narrowed, and the flush of anger crossed his pleasant face. I had intruded on his territory; he was the authority. Since he had no medical knowledge, he tried a different tack. "Well, there's no sense hauling her around. Even if she got better, she might get hit again—or killed during the hunting season. There's plenty of deer out here."

That did it. I was no longer halfway cool. "What the hell kind of sense does that make? You want to kill her just because she might get killed later! She might *not* get killed later!" I took a deep breath. I was shouting, but I couldn't help myself. "I'll take care of her. You don't have to do anything!" I scooped up the fawn and headed for the Bronco. Over my shoulder, I called in a more civilized tone of voice, "Thanks for calling, Mr. Simmons."

Gently I placed the fawn in the back of the Bronco. Then I headed for the hospital.

Tenille was accustomed to wild animals. She gave the new patient a brief sniff and looked at me with those golden eyes, as if urging me to hurry.

"I'm hurrying." I smiled at Tenille. "We did the right thing back there, didn't we?"

Tenille wagged her tail twice and began licking my face.

Of course we had done the right thing. No doubt about it!

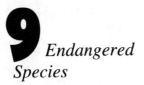

9 Endangered Species

Species in Wisconsin are categorized by the Department of Natural Resources in accordance with their relative population numbers in the wild. There are four groups.

The category to which most species belong is known as "abundant." Obviously this group is doing well as a species.

Next comes the "watch" list, which identifies those species that require close surveillance. Placing a species on this list means that a problem with the wild population may be imminent, though none is identifiable at the moment.

The "threatened" list includes those species whose numbers are declining; this group may be in danger of dwindling further.

The Wisconsin "endangered" list includes those species and subspecies that are in danger of being wiped out entirely.

Most of my wildlife patients fell in the abundant category for obvious reasons; the more plentiful the species the more likely that they should be injured. When presented with a mammal or bird other than abundant, I found myself under greater pressure to save the patient.

The first endangered patient I ever treated was an immature bald eagle. I called him Ernie.

Ernie was a victim of a rare northern Wisconsin storm that produced winds of ninety miles an hour. Ernie had literally been blown from his nest. When he crashed to the ground, his right shoulder was dislocated. A forest ranger found him and delivered him to my clinic one summer afternoon.

"Good God!" I exclaimed when I saw him. "He's not even full grown, and look at the size of him!" The immature eagle stood at least two feet high!

Ernie's head and tail, rather than being white like those of his parents, were a dusky brown, and some white showed on his breast and on the underside of his wing feathers. He was, indeed, an impressive sight.

Suddenly I felt charged with responsibility. Awed, I placed Ernie in one of the dog runs and set a few logs inside to make him feel more at home. Then I tossed in some fish. He ate them all, adapting to his confinement in good order.

Radiographs confirmed what I had suspected in my initial examination of Ernie. Yes, the fall from his nest had dislocated his shoulder. Replacing dislocated shoulders in birds is tricky business. Since I'd never done it or even seen the surgical procedure, I sent Ernie off to my good friend Dr. Pat Redig at the University of Minnesota. Since bald eagles were on the endangered list, I felt that this was no time to attempt a new and difficult procedure. Anyway, my hospital lacked the facilities for the extended hospitalization Ernie would require.

As I had hoped and expected, Pat repaired Ernie's shoulder successfully. After four months of hospitalization, Ernie was returned to the wild in good form.

I had treated two other bald eagles during my first couple of years in wildlife work. Both were mature eagles with regal white heads and tails, magnificent creatures. In both instances, after providing emergency treatment, I sent them off to Pat Redig where I knew they would receive the best of care. Both eagles had been shot, and I was infuriated to the point of explosion. In both cases, someone had taken aim and fired a gun at a member of an endangered species.

Since it is impossible to confuse a mature bald eagle with any "legal" hunting target, the individuals who pulled the trigger had to know what they were doing. To make the situation

Race Foster and
a mature bald eagle

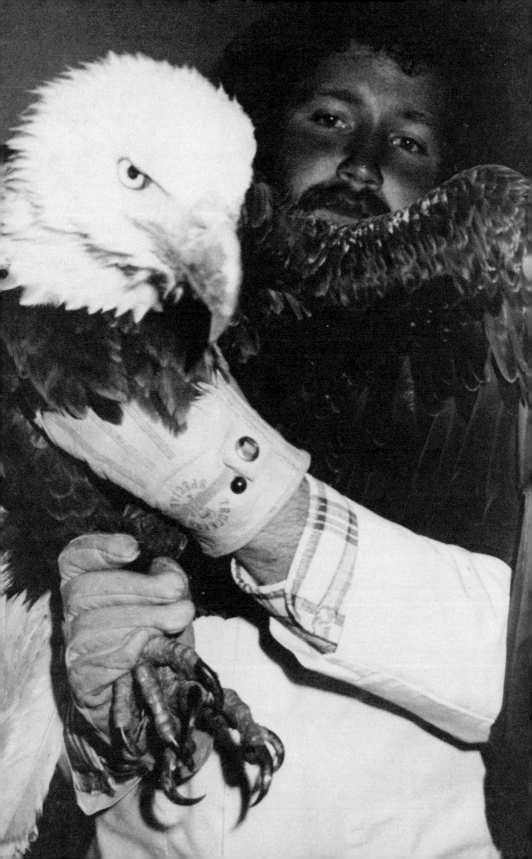

even worse, one of the eagles had been shot in June, when no hunting was allowed.

I lost my first endangered patient in June 1980. It was a week after Tenille and I had picked up the fawn that Dick Simmons had struck with his car.

Race was on vacation from school again. He was assisting me at the hospital when the injured patient was carried through the door by two bearded men.

Karen said, "They've got an osprey wrapped in a sleeping bag."

"Bring 'em into the examining room," I told her. "And tell Race to come on along."

Shortly we were clustered around a loosely rolled sleeping bag, the osprey resting calmly inside. I looked up at the young man standing next to me. He reminded me of one of my roommates in college, wire-rimmed glasses, long hair, and untrimmed beard. "Where exactly did you find the bird?"

"Like, man, we were canoeing down the Manitowish River up near Alder Lake. It's really far out up there. We were just floatin' around some backwaters and saw this bird in the water. So we paddled up to it, and it didn't fly." He nodded to the other bearded young man. "Don here picked it up, and we headed out."

I smiled. He even talked like my college roommate. I turned to the other young fellow. He sported a red bandanna around his neck, and a leather pouch hung from his belt. "That's it?"

"Swear to God," said Don. "That's just how it happened. We took it back to the campground where we're stayin', and some man there told us to wrap it in somethin' and bring it here. Said it was an osprey."

Race reached out and unfolded the sleeping bag carefully. We were all taken aback by the sight of a spectacular mature osprey, nearly as large as a bald eagle. Though I had never seen an osprey before, I'd studied enough pictures of them to know one on sight.

The soft ivory-white underside, dark brown back and flight feathers, and brown masklike coloration of the face distinguished the powerful creature from its relatives. As in all the descriptions I'd read, the legs were heavily muscled, and the feet carried long, razor-sharp talons. "Magnificent" was the only word that would describe the bird!

My first clinical observation went something like this. "It's unable to stand. Place a log under it, Race."

Race went for a log. When he returned, he carefully slipped the log beneath the osprey.

"That's odd," I said. "Its feet didn't even open when you stood it up."

I turned to the canoers. "Did this bird try to strike you with its feet when you picked it up?"

Don wrinkled his brow, thinking.

"Well?" I prodded him.

"No, sir," Don said finally. "Come to think of it, that bird didn't try to claw us or nothin'. Swear to God, he didn't struggle at all. Seemed almost glad to see us."

"In that case," I told them, "you guys can go back to canoeing. This bird has some serious problems. We'll have to take X-rays and do some tests. But I do appreciate you bringing it in."

Don shook his head. "Far out, man! A wildlife doctor!"

The canoers thanked me and moved on out.

When the door closed, Race laughed and said, "Were those guys a little spaced out or what?"

"Reminds me of the sixties," I said as I turned my full attention to the osprey. "He's among the endangered," I added.

"Yeah," said Race.

"Since you've had all those avian courses, maybe you can tell me what the hell is wrong with this bird."

Race pinched one toe of the osprey very hard. The osprey didn't feel a thing; it didn't move.

"Well," I pondered, "if it can't feel down there, then

something must be wrong with the spinal cord. Did you notice? It hasn't moved its wings either. Maybe it's got some kind of neck injury.''

Race nodded. ''But what could have happened to an osprey's neck? Now that's a question.''

I thought back over the six or seven neck injuries I'd treated in birds. Two of them had been shot, and the other four or five had flown into something. ''Remember that sharp-shinned hawk that hit the radio antenna last year?''

Race remembered. ''But there's not much to fly into where the osprey was found.''

''True,'' I admitted. ''Maybe he's been shot. Let's see.''

Together we began picking the osprey's feathers apart in search of a gunshot wound. Since an osprey's feathers are thick, slight bleeding from a shotgun wound might not be easy to detect. But in time we found it.

''There,'' I said. ''Here's the hole.'' I pointed to a tiny opening in the skin over the breast muscle.

''And here's another one,'' Race said. ''Look. It's near the base of the skull.''

''Damn, some ass shot it!''

Aggravated beyond telling, we transferred the osprey to the radiology room for a full set of body X-rays. While Race performed that chore, I hurried into my office to scan my bird books—subject: ospreys.

Ospreys are unique in the hawk world, I learned. They have a reversible outer toe for catching fish and a nostril they can close at will, clear adaptations to their method of fishing, evidenced by the osprey's terrific feet-first plunge from heights of as much as three hundred feet. The osprey hits the water with tremendous force, often submerging in search of fish. Because Wisconsin had only about 138 active nests at that time, the osprey was listed as an endangered species.

Several factors were involved in the fast disappearance of the osprey. Reproductive problems had resulted from the pesticides used during the 1950s and 1960s. There had been a reduction in suitable nesting habitats. Ospreys like to nest in very high places, perhaps a lone dead tree or a utility pole, and forestry practices had removed most of the old dead trees from the areas in which the osprey lived. I didn't have to read further on the subject of threats to the species, since Race came in with the osprey's X-rays.

Our osprey had three shotgun pellets in its breast, one in its thigh, and one in the brainstem at the base of its skull. "Well, what do you think?" I said, as I studied the X-rays up against the viewer.

"The ones in the breast and thigh are no problem. But I figure the one in the brainstem is causing the paralysis. Looks to me like it's not going to make it. Maybe it'd be more humane to put it asleep."

"Asleep?" I exploded. "There are only a few ospreys left in the entire state of Wisconsin. I can't put it to sleep!"

"It's not your fault, Rory." Race was the voice of reason. "Maybe it'd just be better if—"

"No! You know that some people are opposed to our program. What if it got out that I had killed off a member of an endangered species?" I turned away from the X-rays to check on the osprey. Race followed me up. But we were too late.

Already the osprey was having muscle tremors of the head and neck. This was followed quickly by a fifteen-second convulsion. Then it died.

For at least a minute neither of us spoke. Finally Race shook his head and said, "How could anybody shoot a bird as beautiful as this?"

"I don't know." My voice sounded as helpless as I felt. I walked away to stare out the window, contemplating the irony of life. I shrugged and said, "Remember how we thought the guys who brought the osprey in were—well, weird?"

"Yeah."

"Well, the guy who shot that osprey probably looks and talks like most people we know. If that person came in here with a dog, we'd probably think the bastard was normal!"

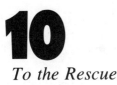

10
To the Rescue

It was November 1975 when I met Marty Smith at Iowa State University in Ames. Marty was a senior veterinary student; I was a newly arrived resident in the department of small-animal medicine. I had traveled to Iowa State after a year of private practice in Rhinelander, Wisconsin, with expectations of completing a three-year residency leading to board certification in the specialty of internal medicine. At that time, I thought I might like to teach at one of the nation's veterinary colleges.

Marty, a tall, lanky fellow, was a couple of years older than I was. He had short, curly hair, a large, slightly hooked nose, and he wore glasses. When I first saw him, I thought he was in the wrong building. I thought he should have been over in Egerton Hall with the engineers or in Bailey Hall with the accountants. But it wasn't long before I realized he belonged right where he was—in Stange Hall, the veterinary college.

Marty was one of the top students in his class. Occasionally he was a bit cocky, and he seemed more mature than his classmates, but I attributed that to a four-year stint in the army prior to veterinary school.

Oddly enough, while Marty and I were striking up a friendship, Linda and Marty's pretty wife, Judy, were working together in the veterinary college admissions office. Unknown to us, they, too, had become friends. Our friendship, it seems in retrospect, was meant to be.

Linda and I began seeing Marty and Judy socially. The four of us got along just great. In fact, the most memorable evening Linda and I enjoyed in Ames was with the Smiths—February 27, 1976, the day Linda and I were married.

Marty and Judy picked Linda and me up at our apartment at 7:19 P.M. I was in a rush. "We're supposed to be at the attorney's office at seven-thirty sharp," I reminded Marty from the back seat of the car.

"No problem," Marty assured me. "I'll get you there on time."

From that point on, Marty gave it all he had, whipping in and out of traffic until we were two blocks from our destination. Here he began swearing profusely at a train that blocked our path. "Damn, damn, damn! This could take forever."

"We don't have forever," I reminded him.

He waved a hand. "Yeah, I know. . . . Hold it. I remember another way!" Marty slammed the car into reverse, backed up a few feet and made a sharp U-turn. "There's a road under the track a few blocks down the street."

Five minutes later at exactly 7:32, we arrived at attorney Ben Hutchin's office. Once inside, we proceeded with the business at hand and departed, fourteen precise minutes having passed. As we came upon the railroad crossing, once again we encountered the still waiting train.

While we sat there, Judy in her customary classy style pulled a bottle of champagne and four glasses from beneath the seat. She filled the glasses and passed them around.

As the red and white caboose came into sight, Marty proposed a toast: "To Linda and Rory—we wish you many happy years together!"

A few weeks later Linda and I made the decision that would affect us throughout our lives. We decided to forgo a career in academia and return to Wisconsin's north woods to start a practice in Minocqua, the small town twenty-five miles northwest of Rhinelander. Our friendship with the Smiths, though, didn't end there.

Four years later in June 1980, Marty left a practice in Madison, Wisconsin, and joined me as a partner in Minocqua. Although he had gained much experience through his small-animal practice in a busy city, it was his enthusiasm for wildlife medicine and surgery that had helped make the decision to join me.

Marty and I had been practicing together for one month when, on a sunny July day, he answered the telephone to hear a woman demand, "Is this the wildlife joint?"

"This is the Northwoods Wildlife Hospital," said Marty. "We don't have an actual wildlife hospital yet, but this is its temporary headquarters."

"I ain't gonna be charged, am I?"

"Normally we don't charge for wildlife care," Marty said. "What's the problem?"

"There's this heron—a blue heron, I think. I've been watchin' it from my window for nearly a week. It just stays in one spot by the small island out in the lake. Never moves. It's gotta be injured."

"Can you see any sign of an injury?"

"Of course I can't," the woman shot back. "Not from here. It's out in the lake. I've been coming up to this cottage for nineteen years. I've seen plenty of herons out there. But they never just stay in one spot. It must be injured. This is the place that helps injured wildlife, isn't it?"

"Okay, okay," Marty said smoothly. "I'll come out tonight after appointments and take a look."

Since I'd made no plans for that evening, I joined Marty on his drive to the lake. We arrived around eight o'clock at the woman's cottage. From her yard we could see the great blue heron standing among the bullrushes and water lilies near a small tree-covered island.

"This is the seventh day it's been standing right there," the woman said. "I'm positive it can't fly." She pointed to an old wooden rowboat tied to a dilapidated dock in front of her cottage. "Why don't you take my boat and have a closer look?"

We were dressed in shirts and ties, but we were willing. We climbed aboard the twenty-foot antique boat to make the trip

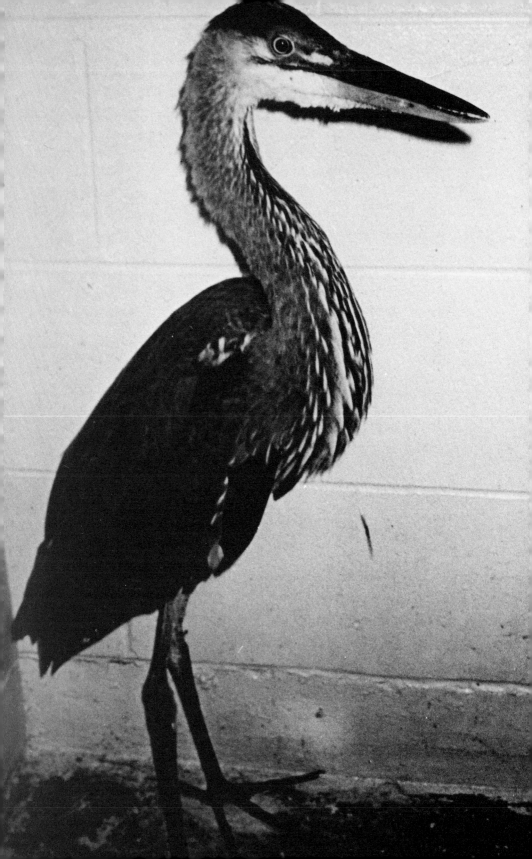

to the island about two hundred yards away, Marty sitting in the bow. He said, "I'll catch the bird. Just get me close enough to grab him."

"Why don't you row? I'll catch him," I said. "Remember, this is *your* call. I'm just here to watch an expert in action."

"No, Foster, you row." Marty could be high-handed. "I've had great experience with these birds. I did banding of blue herons with the Audubon Society while I was in school in Maryland. I know how to handle them. You don't."

Such bull! "I don't want to hear it," I groused. But I began to row the waterlogged boat.

With each stroke the rowing became more difficult as the oarlocks squeaked loudly.

"Foster," Marty said, "row faster. It's going to get dark on us."

"Look," I said testily, "if you don't like the way I'm rowing, *you* row."

"No, no. You're doing just fine. But try to pick up the pace a bit!"

My shoulder muscles were aching as we approached the island. Despite the grinding noise of the oars, the tall bird didn't move.

"Maybe," said Marty, "if you row right up to it, I can grab it."

Since this sounded like a reasonable approach to the problem, I eyed the thirty-foot expanse between us and the heron

A young blue heron stands in the dog run at the Foster-Smith Animal Hospital. Rehabilitating blue herons eat several pounds of fresh fish daily, providing a good excuse for someone on the staff to go fishing each day, usually the author.

and took up my chores again, rowing until we came to a thudding halt. The heavy boat had hit bottom. Forward movement was beyond the scope of our talents. Since it was growing dark, we had no choice but to pursue the bird on foot.

"Foster, go get him," Marty directed, as if I were some sort of elegant bird dog.

"What?"

"Fetch!" said Marty.

"I refuse. You're the expert on herons. *You* go get him. Enough's enough."

Marty mulled it over for a few moments.

"Damn it, Marty," I said, growing irritated now, "go grab the bird before it gets dark. There aren't any lights on this boat."

Marty eyed me balefully. "No fetch?"

"No fetch," I said firmly.

Very reluctantly Marty removed his shoes and socks; then he stepped overboard. The soft, silty bottom gave way under his two-hundred-pound frame; with each step he sank deeper and deeper, until he was in over his knees. "Foster," he proclaimed, "this is ridiculous. What are we doing out here?"

"The blue heron," I reminded him.

"Oh, yeah, the blue heron." He lurched onward through the bullrushes toward the bird. When only a few feet away from the great blue heron, the bird gave a shattering, startling cry loud enough to wake the dead, leaped upward and flew to the far side of the lake and out of sight.

Marty stood there in thigh-deep murky water. His light blue shirt and striped tie were splattered with gray mud. His face was sour. "This ain't gonna cut it, Foster."

I smiled at him from my safe perch in the boat, holding the oars. "Tough," I said.

Just then a yellow canoe rounded the far tip of the island, heading our way. Under the circumstances, I didn't want to meet anyone I knew. I slumped low in the boat, covering my face with my hand and turning away from the oncoming canoeists. My ridiculous companion, however, had no place to hide.

As the canoe drew near, one of the two occupants said, "Is that you, Dr. Smith?" The man's uncertain tone of voice left no doubt that darkness and a settling fog made positive identification impossible.

Through my fingers, I peeked at my partner. Oh, no, I thought: How in the world was Marty ever going to explain this? Getting caught out here in such a predicament would only serve to confirm what many local residents already thought of us— that the doctors who ran the wildlife program weren't playing with a full deck.

But Marty straightened to the task, valiant and inventive to the bitter end. In a thick German accent, he said, "You must ze wrong person haff. Schmidt I am not!"

"Oh, sorry," the man called out. "I thought you were my vet." The canoe passed on, away from us.

"Get into the boat, you nut!" I ordered.

"Ach," said Herr Doktor Schmidt, "I vass plannink to do just that!"

The next week I drove back to the lake. Sure enough, our friendly blue heron was standing in exactly the same spot. Our unwelcome evening visit to his favorite fishing hole had not upset him as much as it had Herr Doktor Schmidt, the noted blue heron expert.

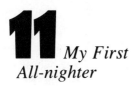 *My First*
All-nighter

All-night monitoring of critically ill dogs or cats is a fairly common procedure in veterinary practice. Many times during my first two years of small-animal work, I was forced to keep an all-night vigil with a canine or feline patient. Finally, I decided to set up a cage and treatment area at home to avoid repeated trips back to the hospital to check on a sick or injured pet. This was much more convenient, because quite often I was able to persuade Linda to check for me, giving me a few hours of uninterrupted sleep.

All-night vigils with wildlife patients are rare, however. Usually, if an injured bird or mammal makes it to the hospital, it doesn't require around-the-clock care. Of course, there are exceptions, and a spectacular bald eagle named Trapper was the first wild patient I kept an all-night vigil with.

Trapper arrived at the animal hospital late on a snowy October evening, brought to me by one of the area's best-known trappers, Bill Sanders.

Bill, a short, thin man about forty-five years old, had a thick stubble of whiskers that never progressed to a beard. I figured Bill shaved about once a week and let it go at that.

Bill's only source of income was trapping; he was a member of a dying profession, one of the last of his breed. He never made much money at it, but his income was enough for him. He didn't need the frills of life. Word had it that Bill owned only one set of clothes. When they wore out, he purchased a new outfit.

His uncomplicated life-style was reflected most dramatically in his cabin. He didn't have running water or electricity.

Under usual circumstances I wouldn't have had a chance to see it. But when the parvo virus epidemic of 1980 hit the north woods, it seemed practical to pay him a house call to vaccinate his dogs—all seven of them—rather than have him haul the whole pack into the clinic. Anyway, it would be a pleasant respite from the hustle and bustle of the clinic.

Bill lived alone about twenty-five miles north of Minocqua near the Upper Michigan border in one of the wildest and most rugged areas remaining in Wisconsin. After a leisurely drive through the woods past countless lakes, I arrived at a gravel driveway where a yellow sign, chipped and peeling, told me that this was where Bill Sanders lived.

The long, winding driveway was lined with glistening white birch trees with a few scattered pines thrown in at irregular intervals. All of it was pristine and natural. About a quarter of a mile in, Bill's log cabin sat next to a small lily-covered pond. It was a picturesque scene, but I reminded myself I wasn't here to enjoy the scenery. I had to vaccinate Bill's dogs and get on back to town.

When Bill opened the door to my knock, his seven canine companions bolted in front of him and barked in unison at my intrusion. Their owner, dressed in patched and faded blue jeans and an equally faded red plaid flannel shirt, stood grinning from ear to ear. His left cheek bulged with an enormous wad of tobacco.

Bill spat and said, "Come on in, Doc. Never mind them dogs. They're friendly."

I took my chances and followed Bill into the cabin. "You got a nice place here," I yelled conversationally above the din of the barking.

Bill hushed the dogs, grinned, and said, "You wanna go fishin' first or you wanna give the shots? There's some big bass out there." He pointed in the direction of the pond.

"Fishing?" I stepped back. "Oh, no, Bill, I can't go fishing. I have an appointment at the hospital in less than an hour."

"Okay, okay. You city folk are always hurryin' somewhere. Let's do the dogs."

I couldn't help but like Bill Sanders. He didn't have much in the way of worldly possessions, but he took good care of his dogs, all of which had once been strays. Local residents knew his soft spot and tied unwanted dogs at the end of his driveway, knowing he'd find a place for them in his heart. Each time that happened he brought the animal in for vaccinations and a checkup; but he always stood in the examining room while I worked, cussing the folks who'd leave a dog like that, while stroking his new companion gently.

Now Bill closed the door behind me and for the first time I took a good look at the interior of the cabin. Dog hair covered the wooden floor almost like a carpet. The faint odor of dog urine permeated the air. Over in one corner was Bill's bed, with four Planters Peanut cans on the floor beside it. On closer inspection, I realized they served as spittoons, as did the two rusty cans that stood near a rocking chair and by the wooden table.

Bill beamed. "Like it, huh?"

"Oh, sure. Very nice, Bill." I got down to business. "Now for the dogs."

Bill restrained each of his pets, while I gave them the parvo vaccine. I vaccinated Duke and Bear, then Blizzard, King, and Duchess and finally Tanya and Katie.

"Big bass out in the pond, huh, Bill?"

"Yep. Whoppers!"

"I'd really like to go fishing with you sometime. But I can't, not today."

"They's huge, Doc. You just let me know when, and we'll go."

I finished up and packed my kit. "Well, I guess I better be off."

"Thanks for comin' out."

I thanked Bill for letting me come out. While the cabin left much to be desired, the environment was superb.

The next time I saw Bill was on that snowy October evening when he came into the clinic. Almost immediately I sensed that something was very wrong. His weatherbeaten face was downcast and somber. Tobacco bulged in his cheek, as usual, and he wore the same plaid shirt and jeans, but they were much more faded and carrying several new patches.

"Something wrong with the dogs?" I asked. "You look upset."

"Well, not exactly."

"Is there anything I can help you with?" I was concerned for Bill, and he seemed strangely reticent.

For a long moment, he said nothing. Then, one eye started to twitch uncontrollably, and his upper lip quivered. "Doc," he blurted out, "you gotta help me."

"Fine. But you have to tell me what you want. Come on, Bill, what is it?"

He glanced around the room. "Anyone else here in the hospital?"

Mystified, I said, "No. I'm here alone. Why?"

More silence. Then: "I caught an eagle this morning in one of my traps, Doc. I let her out, but she couldn't fly. So I took her back to my cabin, thinking maybe she'd be better in a while. But she still can't fly. Maybe she broke a wing or somethin'. I don't know what's wrong. I've been worried sick all day."

I felt somewhat relieved, though not much. "Why didn't you bring her on in, if you've worried all day?"

"Hell, I didn't want nobody to know I caught her in a trap. I got problems enough as it is without all those anti-trapping fanatics on my back."

That was plain enough. "Where's the eagle?"

"In my truck. But you gotta promise you won't tell anyone it was me that caught her in my trap."

I promised.

Bill tugged at my sleeve. "Come on, then. Let's see what we can do for her."

As we walked out into the snow to Bill's truck, I wrestled with the thought that it was my duty to record the person who had found the injured bird. But I decided against it. I'd promised.

The snow fell silently around us. Already Bill's truck tire tracks to the front door of the clinic had disappeared. Inside the truck, he retrieved the bird, which he had wrapped in a burlap sack. We took it inside, bag and all.

Once we'd stamped our feet and warmed up, I carefully unrolled the burlap sack to remove the exhausted eagle. I'd treated three bald eagles in the past, but no matter how many I saw, their spectacular appearance never ceased to amaze and awe me.

Bald eagles don't don their distinctive white color before age four. So when I saw her white head and tail, I knew she had to be at least four years old. Beyond that, I didn't have a clue, since many eagles live to be fifty. I described her on my chart as "mature," meaning somewhere between four and fifty.

As I bent over the exam table, preparing to go over the eagle, Bill said suddenly, "Doc, I gotta go. I'll just leave her here with you."

I paused, thinking back to my duty, and decided to offer one last bit of advice. My suggestion might not sit well with Bill, but it could prevent another eagle from being caught.

"Bill," I said, "before you go, I just want to mention that birds of prey in this part of the country are strictly sight feeders; they have no real sense of smell. Those meat-baited traps set for mink or raccoon are deadly to these birds. This is the eighteenth hawk, eagle, or owl I've seen this month already. God only knows how many more were found dead in traps, or not brought in." The meat-baited sets were one of the biggest threats to bald eagles in Wisconsin.

Bill was at the door. He turned back abruptly and opened his mouth as if to speak.

I beat him to it. "Bill, I know you're sensitive on the subject of trapping. I used to trap, too. I grew up in a family in

Michigan that had always trapped. Before I went to veterinary school, I trapped with my father, but I have to say I'd never do it again. Just the same, though I don't condone the use of leg-hold traps, I understand your point of view.''

His face flushed a bright and angry red. Then, slowly, the anger faded. Perhaps it was the fact that I'd trapped once upon a time. I don't know. He stretched his hand out to me. I shook it. "Thanks, Doc," Bill murmured, "for everything. I gotta go feed my dogs now." And he disappeared through the door into the silent, thick snow falling.

Satisfied that all was well between Bill and me, I turned my undivided attention to the eagle. The inside toe on its left foot was twice as big as the other digits, obvious evidence of the bite of Bill's steel trap. Except for this, the eagle appeared normal. No fractures palpable. Though the feathers were ruffled farther up the body, I could find no other problem, until I came to the enormous wings.

The eagle lay fairly still on her back as I stretched her wings out. The wingspread topped seven feet across easily. But under each wing, the skin, which should have been yellowish pink, was a dark beet red. If I hadn't become accustomed to seeing trap injuries, I might have thought the eagle had a bizarre skin disease. But I knew what had happened here.

The frantic victim, once caught, had tried in vain to escape. The endless hours of beating and flailing her wings had damaged and inflamed the tissue, resulting in the deep red color. Many birds of prey captured by a trap struggled until they died.

Even though the bald eagle population in Wisconsin numbers only in the hundreds, several are brought to the clinic each year for treatment. This one was treated for a blood infection which was induced by a leg-hold trap.

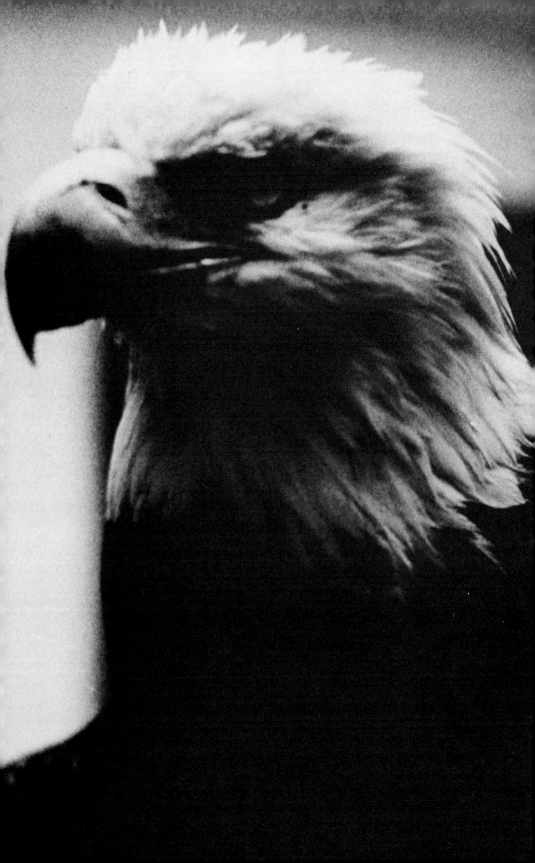

This eagle was smarter—or perhaps she had been found before death caught up with her.

I radiographed both wings, both legs, and the rest of Trapper to check for other injuries. I could find none. Trapper was just plain physically exhausted. She made no attempt to fly. In fact, she could barely stand.

To strengthen her and prevent her from going into shock, I began intravenous infusion of Lactated Ringers, a plasma-like solution, and gave her antibiotics and steroids. The steroids combat stress—a poorly understood but potentially fatal syndrome in wild birds abruptly introduced into captivity.

By 10:00 P.M., Trapper hadn't improved. I repeated the injections. Then I left the hospital, heading for a local fish store to purchase fresh fish, hoping to tempt Trapper with food she knew and loved.

When I returned, Trapper was still too tired to be interested in eating—even fish, her favorite. I decided to force-feed her. Here was going to be the neatest trick of the week.

Grasping a small section of fish with a hemostat in one hand, while prying the massive beak open with the other hand, I forced the fish past the opening to the trachea, far enough down her throat to stimulate the swallowing reflex. Trapper didn't mind; she didn't seem to care about anything. Evidently she was feeling so hopeless that it didn't make much difference to her. I didn't give up, though.

I kept feeding her from time to time. By midnight she seemed no better. If anything, she was worse. Her eyes were only half open, and when I placed a log in her cage, she didn't have the strength to stand. I propped her up, but she toppled right over. Oh, God, I thought, she's going to die on me. A chill swept over me; I hated losing any patient, but Trapper was special, and a bald eagle to boot. Losing her would be catastrophic, a real personal defeat. She was magnificent and rare, and I wanted her to live.

Once more I opened the cage doors to check her. "Listen, you beautiful creature," I told her, "you're not going to die on me. You hear that? I'm going to make you well." But the question was *how?* The word screamed in my head.

Perhaps I had missed something in my examination. Yes, that had to be it. I rushed back to the X-ray room and went over the films carefully.

Nothing.

I went back to stand and stare at Trapper, searching the memory banks of my mind for something, anything that might turn the tide.

It had been four hours since the last intravenous feeding. I hooked her up again and began a slow I.V. drip. Then I sat down to wait, eyeing her cage all the while. By 4:00 A.M. she seemed a bit more perky. She could stand on the log now, but not for more than fifteen minutes without losing her grip. I decided to repeat the antibiotics and the force-feeding of fish. That behind me, at 5:00 A.M., I washed my hands and filled the coffee machine.

Four cups of coffee later, I felt a little better, but Trapper didn't. The time had come for some real decision-making.

I went to my desk, picked up the phone, and punched out the numbers.

Finally, after four rings, a not too alert voice answered. "Good morning, Republic Airlines, Rhinelander, Wisconsin."

I took a firm grip on the telephone and said, "This is Dr. Foster. I have a patient who needs to go to the University of Minnesota in the twin cities on the six fifty-seven flight."

"Very good, Doctor. Is the patient able to travel alone or will the patient require assistance?"

"She can travel alone. I'll arrange for a doctor from the university to meet her at the airport and pick her up."

"That's fine, Doctor. And how old is the patient?" the voice inquired.

I smiled to myself as I said, "Well, she's adult. I'm not certain of her exact age."

And her name please?"

"Trapper."

"Mrs. Trapper?"

"Yes, I guess you could say that."

"One more thing, Doctor," the reservation clerk cut in. "For our records, I need to know what medical condition she has."

Here was a toughie. "Ah, she was caught by the toe in a trap." Suddenly I began to laugh, out of control. Perhaps it was the night without sleep, too many cups of coffee, I don't know what. But the reservation clerk wasn't fooled, not for a minute.

"Are you the vet from Minocqua?" she asked suspiciously.

I confessed. "Yeah, that's me. I'm sorry. I have an eagle that needs to go to the University Raptor Center. Can you make room for her this morning?"

"Sure. But I wish you'd told me right away. That wasn't funny!" The reservation clerk was unhappy with me.

I laughed and said, "You're right. I'll never do it again." Well, maybe . . .

Since the roads were slick with snow, travel was hazardous. But never mind. I'd done my best for Trapper, and it wasn't working.

I readied the eagle for the flight and headed for the Rhinelander Airport, twenty-five minutes south, feeling good about the decision I had made. When we arrived at the airport, Republic Airlines took over graciously and flew the injured eagle out at no charge. They were very good about such things, never charging for an injured eagle anywhere in the state.

I waved good-bye to Trapper, knowing she would have excellent long-term specialized care at the Raptor Center under the expert care of Dr. Duke and Dr. Pat Redig. The program at the veterinary college dealt solely with treatment of birds of prey. When it came to caring for injured eagles, Duke and Redig were second to none.

Six weeks later, I received a telephone call from Dr. Redig. "I've got good news for you," he said. "Trapper was very ill for nearly a week. But after that, she improved remarkably.

She was released to the wild again at the bald eagles' midwestern wintering grounds along the Mississippi."

"Great!" I said, a cloud lifting from around my shoulders.

"She's off and flying," said Redig.

I imagined Mrs. Trapper soaring aloft, free as the wind; and my eyes were the eyes of an eagle for a brief interval. As I hung up the telephone, I remembered Bill.

That spring, as Bill and I rowed his heavy wooden boat through the lily pads of his pond, planning to catch some of those big lunker bass, I told him about Trapper.

Bill grinned, obviously grateful to me and to the others who had helped Trapper, and said, "That's right good news, Doc. Right good news!"

And it was.

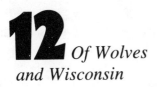

12 *Of Wolves and Wisconsin*

The hospital kennel was uncharacteristically quiet.

I glanced around the room. On my left three cats sat silent in their stainless-steel cages. Nearest the doorway was an eight-year-old tomcat named Benjamin.

Benjamin was a fighter. Even cold January nights didn't slow him down; about every two or three months he ended up in my care as a result. I had just lanced an abscess and sutured a pale yellow tube into his neck so that the wound could drain. Normally Benjamin had lots to say, setting up a fearsome racket when caged. But not today. He sat in the corner of his cage and glared at the center of the room, not at all the fighter I was accustomed to seeing.

Meanwhile, the calico cats in the next two cages might've been in a trance. Both were females who had been dropped off that morning for spaying. They, too, sat low, hunkered over slightly, staring straight ahead.

Nugget, the lone canine patient, hovered in the corner of her run. A golden retriever, she was recuperating from knee surgery two days earlier, but from her appearance one might have thought her days were numbered.

I leaned over and whispered to Nugget, "Don't be afraid."

Nugget stood up, but refused to venture to the front of the run. Only one feeble wag of her tail greeted my overture. Usually Nugget wagged her whole body as a welcome. But Nugget and the three apprehensive felines were foreigners in an alien land.

In the center of the room, inside a wooden-framed wire cage, was a magnificent white Arctic wolf. It wasn't difficult to imagine what she might have been doing if she were in her native habitat. My canine and feline friends seemed to understand this, too. Perhaps their imagination did not soar as mine did. But they knew, yes, they knew.

The ninety-pound white Arctic wolf would have been gliding effortlessly over an unmarked trail in the forests of Alaska. Her graceful movement through the trees would be deliberate and rhythmic, broken only at irregular intervals to check a scent mark along the way or to test the crisp mountain breeze.

By dog standards, the Arctic wolf's feet were massive, a full five inches long. But she would make no sound as she moved. Her powerful, muscular body would appear to float across the frozen ground.

Yes, I could imagine it all. . . .

The northern sun emerges from behind a cloud, striking her pure white two-layered coat. The short, dense fur keeps her warm, even in subzero temperatures, and the long guard hair over the top sheds moisture, breaking the bite of bitter winter winds at sixty below zero. Still she is warm, comfortable, made for this forbidding environment.

Now she stops. A snowy owl is on the ground, clinging to a freshly killed rabbit. And the wolf is off again, never breaking stride, never veering right or left.

Startled by this sudden intrusion, the large white owl flies upward and away, leaving its prey behind, its lunch abandoned. The wolf moves onward, onward along an invisible trail.

Now the wind swirls up from the valley below toward the trail. The smells of spruce and ptarmigan fill the air. The wind twists ever so slightly, and the faint odor of distant caribou crosses her path. She stops to rest. But minutes later her ears come to attention, and she directs her gaze back along the trail behind her. Staring intently, she waits.

Her mate comes into view. His body is larger, more powerful than hers. They meet, nuzzling briefly. Then he turns and heads down the valley toward the caribou. She follows silently.

"Rory? Rory!"

Jolted back to reality, I realized Linda was calling me. I turned around. "Huh?"

Linda stood in the doorway a few feet from me. "What are you doing back here? You look as if you're lost in another world!"

I shook my head and stepped aside. "I was just thinking about her."

"Oh, Rory!" Linda's dark eyes grew wide. "She's gorgeous. I've never seen a white wolf before. Look at those eyes!"

Yes, those eyes. It was impossible to look at the wolf without falling under the spell of her eyes—captivating, cold and distant, farseeing.

Awed, Linda said, "She's the most beautiful animal I've ever seen. But why is she here?"

"She's from Bear Park," I explained. "You know, that roadside wildlife exhibit forty miles south of here. Nothing but a tourist trap. The conditions are terrible. I get complaints about the place all the time. This is a perfect example of their lack of knowledge in animal care."

Linda couldn't take her eyes off of the white wolf. "What happened to her?"

"Last night she got her leg caught in the wire mesh of her pen. The circulation in her leg was cut off, and it was frozen solid. It was thirty-one below last night. You can't tell from the way she's lying. But that right front leg is as hard as a rock."

Immediately Linda wanted to know what we could do.

"Nothing but amputate," I replied glumly. "The leg is frozen past the elbow. If I don't amputate, she'll die."

Linda turned away, demanding, "Where's Marty? I didn't see his car when I drove up."

"He's off today, ice-fishing for walleyes somewhere."

Linda shrugged, glanced back at the wolf, her large blue eyes moist, and said, "I just stopped to give you your lunch. It's in the pharmacy refrigerator. You forgot it *again*." She moved to leave, but her glance was for the wolf. "I have to go. Take good care."

I promised. I didn't miss her point.

As a rule January isn't a very busy month. But this particular morning was different. I was swamped. But at every spare minute I checked on the wolf.

Her unique lack of color had earned her the name Arctic wolf, though she was a member of the same species as other Alaskan timber wolves. But it was her eyes that captivated me—yellow eyes, penetrating eyes—cold. I shivered inwardly as an eerie chill passed through me.

With my other canine patients I could tell by the eyes if the patient was shy or aggressive, friendly or not-so-friendly. But the wolf's eyes told me nothing. And soon I would have to come to terms with her while preparing her for surgery.

That afternoon I faced the inevitable. I hated the thought of the amputation. But past experience with frozen extremities told me it was the only way to save the patient. I had no choice.

Technically, amputation of a front limb is not difficult surgery. But I felt terrible, worse than I remembered feeling in a very long while.

My veterinary practice was for dogs and cats and wild creatures—that is, wild creatures living in the wild. I had no interest in treating captive wild animals, mainly because I suspected that by doing so, I was making myself an accessory to the owner's cruel practice of placing animals on display.

Why work on the animals? I asked myself often. Why? Especially when they'll only return to their tiny cages to be gawked at by thoughtless and uncaring human beings.

Once in a while though, I went beyond my self-imposed restrictions. I had repaired a massive laceration on a captive lynx last year, out of concern for the animal, not for the owner. And so I came to terms with myself about the Arctic wolf. It needed my help, and I would help it.

I began by injecting an anesthetic into the wolf's flank through the wire of the cage. Twenty minutes later she was sound asleep. Gently I lifted her from the cage and carried her into surgery. There I gave her another intravenous injection. Soon she was in a deep sleep, and I stroked her luxurious coat admiringly. Such a beautiful animal.

So that I could monitor her condition during surgery, I clipped the EKG lead into place. The device emitted a high beep with each heart contraction. I could also see each beat on the green oscilliscopic screen located on the emergency cart by the surgical table.

Karen, my surgical assistant, began to ready the leg for surgery.

As I scrubbed for the work ahead, I said to Karen, "What's the heart rate?"

"One hundred ten. Seems steady." Karen paused to lift the upper lip away from the wolf's gums. "The color of the gums is nice and pink."

"Good." This told me much. The color of the patient's gums reveals much about blood pressure in veterinary medicine. The anatomical differences between human beings and four-legged creatures prevented routine monitoring of an animal's blood pressure during surgery. Checking gum color was an accepted substitute. Pink gums indicate good pressure while whitish or lighter pink gums means the pressure is dropping.

At last we were ready, sterile drapes covering the patient except for a small area of humerus directly above the elbow. We sprayed the skin with Betadine solution as a final prep; though Betadine imparted a uniform golden brown to the surgical site, I could see a clear line of demarcation where the leg had been frozen. The skin was turning black from two inches above the elbow. It was now or never.

I made an incision halfway between the shoulder and the elbow, several inches above the area that was going black. Blood spurted up across my glove as I cut through an artery near the surface. I clamped it off quickly and proceeded. Amputations are a bloody mess, I thought to myself. But this was just beginning.

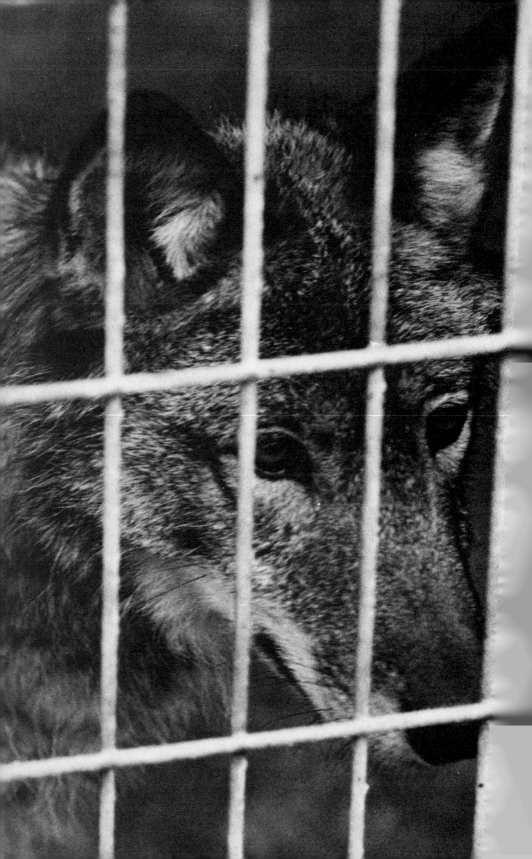

"Heart rate?"

"It's picked up a little," Karen said. "It's one-twenty."

"What's the anesthetic on?"

Karen checked the gas machine. "She's on seven. Want her higher?"

"Seven point five," I said. "And speed up the I.V. fluids. There's quite a bit of bleeding already."

I didn't look up from the surgery. Karen was a fine assistant. She had joined the practice after Linda left to tend to hearth and home. Karen was good at her job, and she was especially reliable during surgery. I knew she carried out my instructions with accuracy, care, and concern.

The razor-sharp scalpel sliced through the lean shoulder muscles. With each deeper cut, the bright red blood oozed from the tissue and into the surgical field. I tied off as many bleeders as I could find and applied pressure on the muscle mass when the blood seeped from everywhere. And all the while I silently cursed the circumstances that had made the amputation necessary.

Now it was time to saw through the bone. I couldn't keep my thoughts to myself a minute longer. "This whole case makes me boiling mad!" I exploded to Karen. "It's so senseless and unnecessary." I glanced up at Karen. "You know who's fault this is?"

Karen nodded wearily. "Russel Borchard. He's the owner, isn't he?"

"He's the owner." I stopped myself before I said something truly tasteless about the man.

The bone made a loud cracking snap as it broke into two pieces.

A mature timber wolf stares
mournfully from its wire cell
in a Wisconsin roadside zoo.

"He should've confined her properly," Karen said then.

"There's more to it than that," I muttered. "Some of the blame goes to the insane Wisconsin law that allows someone to live-trap this wolf last summer in Alaska and sell her to him in the first place."

"That's the truth."

"Then you've got those people who patronize these places and thus perpetuate the cruelty. If they only knew what the poor animals go through. They just pay their money, marvel at the wildlife, and go on. If only people would see the animals' side." And on and on I droned throughout surgery, laying the blame at the feet of those to whom it belonged.

Ninety minutes passed before I had placed the last suture in the skin. Except for the missing leg, the patient looked good. The blood pressure and other vital signs appeared normal. The surgery was a success. The wolf would recover to live again in its cage.

Later that afternoon the wolf was up, standing on three legs, teetering a little from the lingering effects of the anesthetic. True to form, she masked the injury with instinct and effort to stand, just as if nothing were wrong. The wild nature of the wolf prevailed; not even the cold expression in her eyes had changed.

The following morning the owner came to pick up his wolf. Despite the no smoking policy in the office, he paid his bill with a lighted cigarette dangling from his lips.

"Think she'll be all right?" he asked then.

I hesitated. I was having difficulty controlling my emotions. "The surgery went fine," I allowed in as even a tone of voice as I could manage. Then I watched through the office window as he and an employee loaded the travel cage containing the wolf into the back of his pickup truck. That chore done, they climbed into the cab of the pickup and drove off across the frozen parking lot.

Several times, when the wheels of the pickup hit chunks of ice, the wolf bounced violently upward to crash again to the floor of the cage. She seemed to be unaware of what was happening to her. And in that instant I read the hidden meaning in her eyes.

That beautiful Arctic wolf wasn't alive and well. She had died last summer on the day she was trapped in Alaska.

13 *The Right to Arm Bears*

The next, and last, time I broke my rule about not treating captive wildlife came only ten weeks after my heartbreaking experience with the Arctic wolf, on a Sunday afternoon, April 2.

Stan Lambrutti, the owner of another roadside exhibit in the next county left a call for me with my answering service. I telephoned him.

"Is this the veteran?" the man blared into the phone.

My God, I thought, he can't even say "veterinarian" correctly. "Yes, this is the veterinarian," I answered with considerable emphasis on the last word.

"I got this bear cub with diarrhea," Lambrutti blared onward. "He's throwing up all over the place, too, and there's blood in it. He's real weak, Doc. I really wanna save him."

Perhaps I had misjudged the man. "Why?" I asked curiously.

"Got him sold."

Wrong again. "Okay, bring him over to the clinic. I'll meet you there. But just so there's no misunderstanding, our free care to wildlife applies only to animals living in the wild, not to those owned by someone."

That didn't deter him. An hour later I met Stan Lambrutti at the hospital. He was a short, thin guy and very talkative.

"Well, here he is, Doc. His name is Andy." He placed the eight-pound patient on the table.

Andy was my first black bear patient. Speckles of foamy blood were visible around his mouth and chin. "Did he vomit on the way here?"

"Yeah, three times. Looked like pure blood. He had diarrhea, too. It was black."

I checked Andy's rectal area; dark, tarlike, odoriferous stool was smeared into his hair. "The dark color is from blood higher up in the intestinal tract," I told Lambrutti. "It turns black by the time it gets out. How old is Andy?"

He pulled a small notebook from his back pocket and began leafing through it. "Let's see now. Here it is. Andy was born on January twenty-second." He scratched his head. "No, that's wrong. It was the twenty-fourth. Well, wait. That might be wrong, too."

"It doesn't matter," I said, anger growing. "I just wanted his approximate age."

Lambrutti glanced at me with pale eyes. "No, Doc. You got my curiosity up. I'll find it." He continued flipping pages in the notebook. "Ah, here it is. Andy was born on January twenty-ninth. His mother's name is Henrietta."

I continued my examination. The cub's skin felt thick and lacked flexibility. When I picked up the skin over the back, it snapped back slowly, too slowly. Andy was dehydrated to an alarming extent. "How many bears do you have?" I had turned warm and charming, with motive in mind.

"Six adults and seven cubs."

I took Andy's temperature. "Six adults and seven cubs! Boy, that's a lot of bear. What do you do with all those bears?"

"The adults are breeding stock. We sell the cubs each year."

"How about that!" I was enthusiasm itself. "Who buys the cubs?"

"Roadside exhibits. You know, like the ones around here. But mostly I sell to the ones downstate."

"Aren't these bears a bit dangerous as they grow older?" I knew very well how dangerous they were.

"Not usually," Stan said. "See, we take 'em away from their mothers after a few days and raise 'em on a bottle. That way they stay tame for a while."

I removed the thermometer. "Temperature's one-o-four.

That's pretty high.'' I wasn't sure what was normal for a bear, but I was sure that it wasn't 104 degrees. ''Guess you'd better leave Andy here. He's really sick. He's going to need intravenous fluid and some blood tests. There's a very hot infection in there somewhere.'' Gently I palpated Andy's abdomen.

Andy winced in pain and drew away from me.

''See what you mean,'' the owner said. ''I'll call you in a couple of days to check on him.''

''Right,'' I said.

While this owner hadn't proved to be a man one could thoroughly dislike, the business of taking newborn cubs from their mothers was more than a little disturbing to me. It wasn't fair to the mother or to Andy.

This kind of thinking had prompted some people to accuse me of anthropomorphism. But I didn't buy that nonsense. After all, pointing out that a bear has very strong maternal feelings for her offspring didn't make me guilty of attributing human characteristics to bears. The bear's feeling for her cubs was not human; it was bearlike.

I gathered up Andy, now that the owner was gone, and carried him into the surgery room where the lighting was better. His honey-brown face, longish muzzle, and rounded ears made him appear gentle and vulnerable and gave no hint at all that someday, if he lived, he might weigh over five hundred pounds.

Taking careful pains not to hurt the bear any more than it had been hurt already, I made an incision through Andy's skin to find the vein on the front leg, so that I could insert a catheter. So sapped was Andy's strength that he hardly moved at all. Next, I drew blood for routine tests, finally starting him on intravenous fluids. Then I inserted a sterile swab into his colon to obtain a culture; I hoped to identify the organism responsible for Andy's apparent intestinal infection.

Over the next twenty-four hours, I kept Andy on a heating pad and continued fluids along with other medication to combat his weakened condition.

The blood tests indicated that Andy's organs were working

normally. The culture proved helpful, though. A pathogenic bacterium was isolated, and appropriate tests were done to determine the proper antibiotic to combat the bacteria.

On the second day, Andy showed some signs of improvement. I discontinued the intravenous feeding and switched to a bottle. Andy guzzled the formula, and it stayed down. Cheers!

Stan Lambrutti picked Andy up the following day; and that's the last of that, I thought wearily. Then, three months later, on July 6, Marty brought in a Madison newspaper.

"I still get the paper from down there," he explained. "I want you to see this picture of the Fourth of July parade." Marty handed me the newspaper.

I was puzzled. "What for?"

"You know that bear you treated a few months back?"

"Andy?"

"That's the one. Take a look at that picture."

I did; and there was a bear cub in the parade, dressed in Bermuda shorts and a lettered T-shirt. The bear was being led by the paw. "How do you know it's Andy?"

"Look for yourself, underneath the picture."

The caption read: Andy, the bear cub from Treasurewood Animal Land, makes hit at parade.

"Do you really think that's him?" I demanded.

"Could be," said Marty. "How many bear cubs named Andy are there in the state? They sure must have a lot of bears at Treasurewood. That place isn't far from my old practice. Every year they have a cub in the parade."

"Well," I said thoughtfully, "I think I'll just call Treasurewood, in that case, and see if it's Andy." As I was about to pick up the phone on my desk, Marty grabbed my arm.

"Foster, don't blow your stack again. We've made enough enemies with this wildlife stuff already. There's no reason to call that place. You won't accomplish anything, except to make the owner madder than hell. We don't need any more people mad at us."

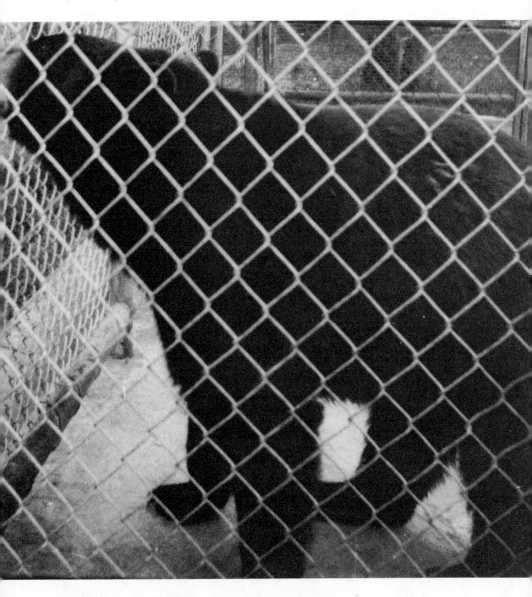

A bear's life in a roadside zoo

Marty made sense. But I was beyond reason. "Okay, okay," I told him.

I waited for Marty to leave my office, and then I placed a call to the roadside zoo.

"Is this the owner?" I asked the man who answered the telephone.

"Yes, I'm Zeb Kowalski. I own Treasurewood."

"I'm calling out of curiosity more than anything else. I'm a vet. I happened to see a newspaper picture of a bear named Andy walking in a Fourth of July parade. I wondered if that might be the bear I worked on for Stan Lambrutti up this way."

"Sure is," Kowalski answered. "I bought Andy from Stan two months ago. He told me Andy'd had an intestinal infection. But there's no sign of it now. He's healthy as they come."

"That's good. I like to follow up on all the patients I treat."

"Well, you did a good job on Andy. Like I said, he's fine."

I sensed the conversation coming to an end. "One more thing, Zeb, as long as I have you on the phone. How many bears do you have down there?"

"Just two. Andy and one adult."

"But I thought you had a bear in the parade every year?"

"I do."

Here was the clincher. "What happens to them after the parade?"

"We keep 'em at the exhibit for tourists until Labor Day· then we sell 'em."

"But who would want a bear that age?"

"Lots of clubs or maybe some group planning a bear rc We can't keep 'em around all winter. They cost too muc feed. Besides, we have one adult here. We don't need an ers."

Andy could be headed for a bear roast! I fought back my rising anger and said, "Well, okay. I just called to check on Andy. I won't keep you any longer." I hung up, and Marty walked into my office.

"Well, what'd you find out from your call?" he demanded.

Marty knew me too well. But I feigned ignorance. "Call? What call? You told me not to call."

"Foster," Marty said disgustedly, "your face is beet red. You're mad, right? I knew you'd call. So what did they say?"

"I need a cigarette," I said, shifty as they come. "You got any?"

"Foster, come to your senses. You don't smoke, and neither do I. Where would I get a cigarette?"

"Why don't you run down to the corner drug store and pick up a pack?"

"What corner drug store? Ye gods, Foster, you've become unhinged. Now tell me all about it."

I slumped in my chair and stared at Marty. "That was Andy, all right. And that's the good news. The bad news is—"

"Uh-oh."

"Yes, there's bad news, too. They do have a cub every year in the parade. But they keep only one adult bear. Get the picture?"

"What happens to them?" Now Marty was more than a little interested in Andy's future.

"They sell the cubs to organizations that are planning a bear roast."

"Oh, God . . ." Marty subsided and flung himself into a chair across the room. "It never crossed my mind that—"

"Marty, I worked my tail off on that cub. For what? So he could be dressed up like a human and paraded through town? So he could sit in a hot cage all summer while kids jeer at him and feed him popcorn and soda pop, and then end up on a spit at a bear roast? It's crazy. Then, next winter another cub will be stolen from its mother, and the whole business will be repeated."

"It probably happens all over the north woods," Marty surmised.

"Yeah, a helluva life cycle, huh?"

We sat in silence for a long moment. Then I had the last word. "If another sick cub from one of those places comes to me, I'm going to arrange a different ending." I paused. "A humane ending. Intestinal infections can be fatal."

Marty nodded, hauled himself out of the chair, and departed the office without another word. We'd made a silent pact. No more bear cubs that I treated would end up being roasted.

14

Miracles

The last patches of snow had melted. It was May again. The renewal of life in the north woods was beginning to flourish.

The new barred owls had hatched two months earlier and were venturing out on their own. On a hike through the woods, I found the fledglings perched motionless on logs or stumps. They had left their nests for a few days, trying it on their own, learning to fly, to soar. But nearby the parents were watching, ever vigilant, making certain the fledglings had a chance at survival.

Not all the new additions to the north woods were born at once. The owls had hatched in March, unusually early. The eaglets had pecked their way out of their eggs in early April. Ducks and loons came along later.

The mammals waited for warmer weather, with the exception of the bear, who were born in their cozy dens back in January. Most furred animals, though, waited for May or early June for a first look at their new world.

All of this, the wonder of new life, the miracle, happened year in and year out. Same time. Same place.

Unlike a farm veterinary practice or my dog and cat practice, doctoring wildlife didn't include assisting patients during the miracle of birth. There were no difficult deliveries requiring assistance. Mostly I treated injured wild patients and, of course, orphans. But I was never around when the species had their young. They carried out this mission in secluded forests and hidden nests.

Four years after I began treating wild creatures, though, I received my first wild animal obstetrics case. Like most deliveries in veterinary medicine, it happened at night. But that was where the similarity ended.

Around midnight the telephone rang. I struggled awake to answer, "Dr. Foster here." Then I realized I was holding the telephone upside down. I turned it around and tried again.

The caller was saying, "Hello? Hello? Is someone there?"

"Yes, I think I'm here. This is Dr. Foster. Can I help you?"

"Yeah, Doc. This is Jerry Fergenson. I just hit a doe with my truck. Out here by Lake Shishebogama. I think she might be dead; I'm not sure. But I can see some movement in her belly. Looks like there's something kickin' in there. Must be pregnant."

I sat up in bed, suddenly wide awake. "Are you sure? I mean, it's just not a nervous twitching—"

"No, Doc. I grew up on a farm. There's a fawn in there. I'm pretty sure of that."

"Did you say you were out by Lake Shishebogama?" I was trying to collect my wits now.

"That's right. I'm at a house near where I hit the doe."

"Okay." I was brisk and efficient now. "Get someone to help you get the deer into the back of your truck. I'll meet you at the hospital. I live out the other way, so that'll be faster." I gave him directions before we hung up.

I hurried from bed, dressed in the dark, and Tenille and I ran for the car. As I drove out of the driveway, a startled beaver slapped its tail on the lake in front of the house, disturbed by this late night noise.

Unexpectedly a wave of apprehension swept over me. It would take me approximately fifteen minutes to drive from my home on Lake Tomahawk to the clinic. Perhaps as much as six minutes had passed since the doe was hit, assuming the man had managed to locate a phone in just five minutes. Surely twenty minutes would be too long for the fawn to survive inside its dead mother. If the doe was indeed dead, the fawn would have suffocated in the womb by now.

I tried to put a better face on the matter. I pictured myself arriving at the clinic and finding the doe alive and the fawn healthy.

As I neared the clinic driveway, I saw that the outdoor light in front of the animal hospital illuminated a parked pickup truck. A man leaned over the bed of the truck, looking inside. Something in his posture said it was too late.

I reached over and held Tenille steady with one hand as I slammed on the brakes and skidded to a stop beside the pickup. Then I opened the door of the Bronco and jumped out. "How's it look?" I called out anxiously.

"Not good, Doc. I haven't seen any movement since I got here."

The big doe lay facing the tailgate, her rear legs resting on the spare tire. No mark was visible on her; she might have been sleeping. I touched one of her open eyes. No blink reflex. I tapped harder. Still no reflex. Almost certainly she was dead.

Now for the abdominal area, I thought. I fixed my eyes there for several seconds, looking for signs of movement. No, nothing. Such disappointment.

"Well," I said, turning to Fergenson, "we've come this far. We may as well be a thousand percent sure." I opened the tailgate and pulled the doe partway out. "You grab the rear legs, and we'll take her inside."

With some confusion—I had to unlock the front door—we made it inside and placed the dead doe on the reception room floor. Then I rushed into the first exam room and returned with a scalpel. Quickly I made a slash from the top of her back to the doe's swollen mammary glands below. The cut hair flew several inches to either side under the force of my blade. Another slash, and I was into the abdominal cavity.

The swollen uterus occupied the entire area I'd exposed with the scalpel. One more swipe, and I went through the wall of the uterus. Greenish fluid mixed with blood spurted out and covered the floor. A spotted fawn bulged through the opening.

I pulled it out and wiped the slippery membranes from its head. The fawn's tongue was a deep purple, and there was no movement. I placed my hand hard against the chest. No heartbeat. Exhausted in defeat, I laid the fawn back down on the mother. I looked up at Jerry Fergenson; he had backed away to the door in an attempt to avoid the uterine fluids seeping out still. "Well, we tried."

"I'm sorry, Doc."

"I'm sorry, too. But thanks for trying."

In this moment of tragedy we were uneasy in each other's company. He thanked me again and departed the way he had come.

Disturbed, weary, sad, I straightened and wandered over to a bench in the reception room. I sat down to gaze at the fawn and the doe, feeling bitter. Then, it occurred to me . . . death is a miracle of sorts, too.

15

Flower

My daughter Ali and I were on the pier overlooking Lake Tomahawk one evening when I heard the telephone ringing inside the
house. After the third ring, I suspected Linda was unable to answer it. So Ali and I darted for the basement phone. At three
and a half years old Ali couldn't run very fast. But she tagged
along gamely.

At the other end of the telephone line was a Mr. Becker,
saying, "My wife just hit a fawn by our house. Wanna come
over and have a look?"

"Sure," I responded. "Where do you live?"

"Just off Forty-seven, north on Bear Marsh Road about one
mile. It's the only house on the left, just before the marsh. Oh,
yeah, I called the DNR guys. I think they're comin', too."

After absorbing this unsettling news, I rallied and said,
"You're about seventeen miles from my house. I'll be there as
soon as possible." I hung up the phone, and Ali and I ran up-
stairs to tell Linda.

Linda was just stepping from the shower.

"Someone's hit a fawn. I'm going to check on it. Do you
want to go?"

Up until four months earlier, Linda had gone on every night
call I'd made. But now Ali's little brother, Michael, only four
months old, made it difficult for Linda to participate in wildlife
evening calls.

"Mikie just fell asleep," she said. "He's not feeling very
well today. You and Ali go. I'll stay up, though, in case you
need help later."

I grabbed Ali's hand, and we hurried along to climb aboard the Bronco. Ali loved going on emergency calls with me. She was at that precious age, when a father and daughter enjoy a very special relationship.

Her face was round, with a small, turned-up, freckled nose, and her hazel eyes beamed enthusiasm and energy my way. She especially loved those calls that involved fawns.

Though Ali was accustomed to all types of birds and animals—for a time she had even shared her room with four baby woodpeckers we'd raised together—fawns said it all for Ali. Perhaps she felt that way because we'd raised one or two fawns a year since her birth; or perhaps it was all those nights of falling asleep while her mother recounted the days of Faline. For whatever reasons, Ali was in love with fawns. Fawns were everything.

Now the questions began. "Daddy, what happened to the fawn?"

"It was crossing the road, and a car hit it accidentally, Ali."

"Why'd it get hit, Daddy?"

"The woman driving the car couldn't stop in time. Sometimes animals run right in front of cars and get hit." I took my eyes from the road and looked at Ali. If I had wished for a dream to come true, Ali was it.

"Why do they go in the road, then?" she asked, perplexed.

"Maybe the fawn was following her mommy."

"Then why'd her mommy go across the road, Daddy?"

"She was probably looking for food."

I half expected the next question to be "And why was the mommy looking for food?" but it wasn't.

Briefly Ali slipped into thought. At last, she said, "What are we going to name the fawn, Daddy?"

"I don't know. Why don't you think of a name, Ali?"

"I know." She snuggled closer to me. "How about Faline?"

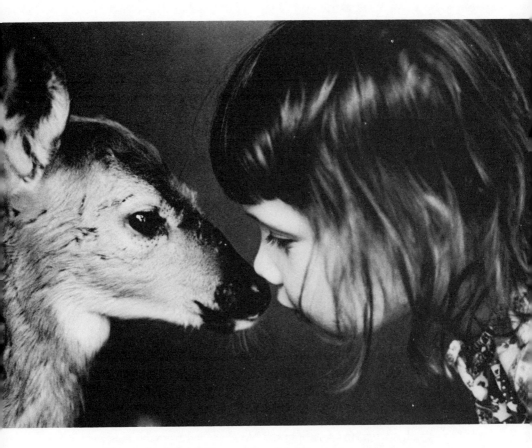

*The author's daughter, Ali, with Blossom, a fawn
that had been hit by a car. Some injured wild creatures
need minimal handling when undergoing medical and
rehabilitative care. This helps to insure that the
patient remains "wild" and capable of successfully
reentering its natural habitat. We found, however,
that the survival rate of injured fawns at the
hospital was directly proportional to the amount
of attention given them. Indeed, like many baby
mammals, fawns thrive on TLC.*

"No. We've already used that name. We need a new name."

"I know." Ali was bubbling now. "Blossom!"

"Silly," I laughed, "we had a Blossom last year."

"Oh, I remember." Ali considered, adding, "I forgot!" She giggled as little girls sometimes do when they forget.

"I've got it!"

"What?" She leaned over, as if we were conspirators.

"How about . . ."

"What, Daddy?"

"Flower!"

"Oh, Daddy, that's wonderful. I like flowers."

And so it was all settled—Flower it would be—as we approached the lights of several vehicles pulled off the road. This had to be the place, and yes, I was right. A dark green DNR truck sat waiting.

A man in a tan uniform walked over to the Bronco. He was tall, rather gaunt, with auburn hair and a small well-groomed mustache. He looked just old enough to have graduated from college.

I told him who I was and why I was there.

"Nothing for you to do, Doc. Looked like the fawn had a broken leg, so I shot her." He pointed his flashlight to the side of the road. Crumpled in the grass just a few feet away was a small spotted fawn. Bright red blood seeped from the bullet wound in her head, and the fawn's tiny nose rested in the pool of blood as it formed beneath her.

Without a word, I fired up the Bronco and drove off down the road, looking for a place to turn around. To say I was bitter would be putting it mildly. I whipped around at a wide place in the road. Three more DNR employees stood there. Did it take four men to kill a tiny fawn? I wondered bitterly. Four men?

As Ali and I headed homeward, the windows down, the sounds and smells of summer off the marsh rushed in to greet us, reminding me of life. Cautiously I glanced over at Ali. Her innocent face was flooded with sadness; the expectation in those big hazel eyes was gone.

What could I say to make it right? Nothing, I guessed. I waited, for surely the question would come.

Finally: "Daddy, why did the man shoot Flower?"

I didn't have an answer for her. Certainly this killing made no sense to me. Though I knew life was cheap to many people, I wasn't prepared to share this fact of life with Ali. Not yet. So, as all good fathers do, I changed the subject. "Hey, Ali, listen to the bullfrogs' croaking. They're out there calling to you in the dark."

But Ali wasn't listening.

We drove home in dreadful silence.

Moose

Moose, a fifty-pound dark brown Plott hound, sat on the stainless-steel exam table waiting for me to remove the hundred or so porcupine quills that were buried deep in his mouth and face. Moose was dejected; his ears hung low, and his head drooped almost to the tabletop, as if the weight of the quills pulled his head downward.

As I prepared to relieve Moose of his agony, I smiled at his identification tag: Moose—Reward if Found—Tom Beamer. I patted Moose's left flank where the letter *B* had been freeze-branded.

Freeze-branding is a technique practiced by some bear hunters in our part of the country. A branding iron is chilled with liquid nitrogen or dry ice and applied to a sedated dog's flank for about twenty seconds. The process freeze-burns the hair follicles, so that when the hair grows in again, it sprouts back a glistening pure white, making identification of the dog unmistakable. During bear-hunting season, dogs occasionally get lost in the vastness of the northern forests while pursuing a bruin for miles and miles. Since a brand is permanent and can't be disguised, it increases the chances of a dog like Moose being returned to its rightful owner. Meanwhile, it's a powerful deterrent to the serious business of hound-stealing.

So Moose was protected by his owner in every way possible; he was a valued dog. As Tom had told me many times, "Moose—he never loses a track."

Now Tom said to me, "Do you realize this is the fourth time in less than a year that I've brought Moose in here with quills?"

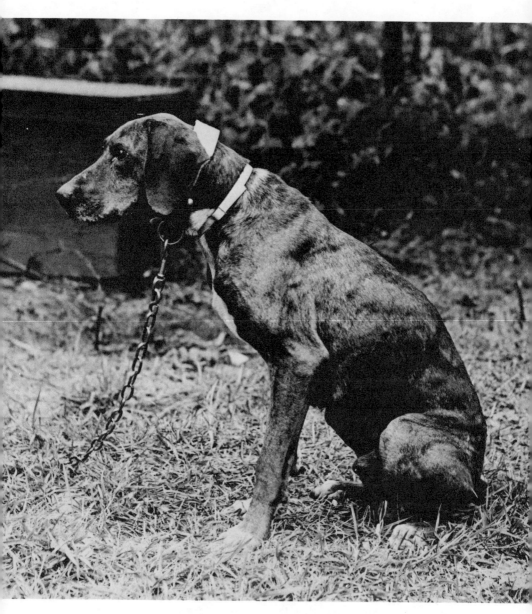

Moose, a Plott hound

"I know," I said.

"It is," allowed Tom, "getting mighty expensive."

"Well, Tom, I don't know what makes some dogs decide to go after porkies. About all you can do is pen him up."

"Those damn porcupines!" Tom fumed. "I'm gonna shoot every goddamn one of 'em I see from now on."

I didn't respond. I had tried to reason with other dog owners on this subject, and I knew how futile it was. Dogs did the attacking, not porcupines. I anesthetized Moose to facilitate the removal of the quills, wishing I could talk some sense into Tom.

Tom Beamer belonged to one of the older clans in the north woods. He was one of the few residents I knew who had actually been born and raised here. At about forty-five years old, he had a bronze complexion that spoke of countless days spent hunting, trapping, and guiding. Local talk had it that the long, jagged scar that started near his hairline and ended above his right eye was the result of having been mauled by a bear. But nobody knew for sure. His family kept to themselves, except when they needed the services of the newcomers.

Slowly Moose sank into oblivion from the anesthetic. I got to work. Removal of the barbed quills took thirty minutes or so. During the entire procedure, Tom groused about porcupines. "What good are they? Just tell me. What good can they do? You can't hunt 'em, you can't trap 'em, you can't eat 'em."

I held my tongue. I sensed there was no convincing Tom that creatures existed in this world for other reasons than benefiting man.

Finally I removed the last quill. After I'd injected a drug to reverse the effects of the anesthetic, Moose began to stir. He sat up sheepishly, glanced around the room, and even managed a friendly wag of his tail, as if to say, Thanks for helping me out!

Moose stayed out of trouble with porcupines for a while after that. But six months later, he was back again, shot full of quills, at least two hundred of the four- to six-inch variety, evidence that he'd attacked a very large porcupine. Ten or so quills were embedded in Moose's tongue, and at least fifty more were lodged in the hard palate on the roof of his mouth and between his teeth. If Moose had been sad before, he was downright mad at the world now. So was Tom Beamer.

Midway through the quill removal procedure, I noticed Tom lingering near the rear of the treatment room, inspecting some of the wildlife patients we had on hand. Our clients enjoyed seeing the wild birds and animals, and Tom was no exception.

"Quite a hawk," he said. "These goshawks, they're really something!"

"Yes, they're a beautiful bird." I pulled a quill from poor Moose. "That one had a broken wing. But it's healing fine now. We plan to release him any day."

Tom peered into the next cage. "What's wrong with this robin?"

Suddenly I felt encouraged by Tom's questions. He seemed interested, genuinely so, in the fate of each wildlife patient. It was a welcome change from most of the old-timers who regarded helping injured wildlife as a frivolous endeavor. "That robin flew into a window this morning," I told him. "Just needs some rest. Then she'll be good as new."

"What about this saw-whet owl?" he asked next.

I marveled at his knowledge of owls. Most viewers didn't know one owl from another. "That one was hit by a car. The impact dislocated his shoulder. We're not sure if it's going to heal correctly or not. He's scheduled for more X-rays later today."

"Do you get all kinds of animals in here, or just birds?" Tom paused, but before I could answer, he asked, "Say, what's in this last cage with the towels covering the front?"

Frequently we covered the cage doors to minimize human contact for patients who seemed upset or might be dangerous to onlookers.

"We get all kinds," I said. But I said no more. In fact, I was holding my breath, because the cage with the towels over it contained a porcupine someone had struck with a car. Tom

would have apoplexy if he found out I was treating one of
Moose's sworn enemies. "Don't look in there!" I cautioned
quickly. "Don't go any closer. There's—ah, ah—a blue heron
in there. He nearly pecked someone's eye out this morning. If
you remove the towels, he'll nail you for sure." Now I decided
to use good old Moose as a diversion. "Tom, Moose isn't
breathing well. His tongue is swollen from the quills. I think
you'd better hold it for me so he can breathe easier."

With that, Tom came running.

"Here," I said. "You just hold his tongue straight out like
this." I placed Tom's hand on the dog's blood-covered tongue.

Tom seemed to forget all about the fictitious blue heron.
"Is Moose gonna be all right?" he demanded.

"That tongue's pretty bad. Now, don't let go. Keep it out
so he can breathe." I spoke in my most professional manner. I
didn't like deceiving Tom, but anything was better than having
him find out that I was harboring an injured porcupine.

"Damn beasts!" Tom groused. "Damn porcupines. I hate
those sonavabitches. Look what they've done to my Moose. I
mean to kill every one I see from here on out!"

If Tom discovered the truth ten feet away, he'd go wild. I
could almost see the newspaper headlines: Local Bear Hunter
Kills Vet and Porcupine.

I pulled out the last quill and injected the anesthetic antag-
onist to awaken Moose. "Ah, I think he's all right now. You
can let go of his tongue, Tom.

"Are you sure, Doc?" Tom was anxious. "What about that
swelling? What about—"

"Don't worry, Tom. The worst is behind us. He'll be fine."
Swiftly I lifted the still drowsy Moose and placed him in Tom's
arms. "Take Moose home and let him rest up for a day or two.
He needs it."

I ushered Tom out to his truck, the epitome of concern.
"Now, don't worry. Moose will be fine. The thing to do is get
him home and let him rest."

Oh-so-gently Tom placed Moose on the seat of his truck

and slid in beside him. He pulled the door closed and said through the open window, "Thanks, Doc. I hope that owl does all right, too."

I smiled, waved, and headed for the front door of the clinic.

"Oh, one more thing," Tom called out to me.

I paused. "What's that?"

"How's that porcupine my neighbor brought in last night?"

"Porcupine?" I croaked.

Tom grinned and winked. "Yeah, the porcupine!"

"He's okay," I replied lamely.

As Tom pulled out of the parking lot, I could hear him laughing fit to be tied. Why, that shameless faker, I bet he'd never shot a porcupine in his life, and what's more, he never would!

17

In Cold Blood

Biologists divide plants and animals into groupings called *phyla*. The *phylum Chordata* includes all mammals, birds, reptiles, amphibians, and fishes.

When I started treating injured wildlife, I thought becoming a wildlife doctor meant treating mammals and birds. About twice a year, though, someone would bring in an injured reptile or amphibian. One day a ten-year-old freckle-faced boy and his mother came into the clinic. The boy was carrying a paper bag; inside the bag was a frog with a fishhook lodged in the roof of its mouth.

"Tell the doctor what happened, Billy," the boy's mother said, pushing the boy forward.

Billy didn't open his mouth; he was on the verge of tears.

I decided to lighten his burden. "Tell you what, Billy. Let's see if I can guess. I'll bet you were walking around the shore on your lake. You were probably going fishing for bass or blue gills. Am I right so far?"

Billy nodded soberly.

"Then you spotted this huge old bullfrog. It was the same frog you'd been trying to catch all summer. But he was too smart for you. Right?"

Billy nodded soberly.

"That frog stayed out on those pads in deeper water, just out of your reach. You didn't want to hurt him. You just wanted to catch him and look at him. Right?"

Billy nodded soberly.

I wasn't sure if I was close to being correct now or if Billy just liked the story I was telling him.

"Today, though," I continued in good form, "you had your fishing pole and worms, and you got an idea. Maybe the frog was hungry. So you put a worm on your hook, leaned out, and dangled it in front of the frog. Right?"

"Right, Doctor." That was the mother. "And can you guess what happened next?"

"The frog jumped up at Billy's bait," I said. "Probably missed it once or twice. Then the frog nailed the bait on the third try and hooked himself!"

"Tell us more," said the mother.

"Well, Billy, you got real scared. You ran back to your cottage with the frog dangling in the air from your pole. You really weren't sure what to do next. But your mom heard the commotion and ran outside. When she saw the frog, I imagine she shrieked once or twice."

"More like six or seven times!" said Mom.

I laughed. "Your dad is probably out on the lake fishing, and your mom wouldn't touch the frog to get him off the line. So you came here. Right?"

Billy had relaxed now. He managed a tentative smile.

"That's almost exactly how it happened," Billy's mom reassured me. "How'd you know, Dr. Foster?"

I winked at the mother. "Let's just say that I used to be your age, Billy, and I did something like that myself once. You know, I even had freckles just like yours. See? They never went away." I pointed to my nose and leaned down so that he could examine my freckles.

At last, Billy grinned.

"Okay, Billy, let's look at your frog."

Billy offered up the paper bag, and I reached inside it to retrieve my cold-blooded patient.

The beast was wiggly, but at long last I got a good grip on him, pulled him out of the sack, and checked him over. The hook was embedded past the barb in the frog's upper lip. "What's the frog's name, Billy?"

"I—I think it's Burt."

"Burt it is, all right!" Poor Burt. "We're not going to be able to put Burt to sleep like a dog or cat. Someone is going to have to hold him while I remove the hook. Do you want to help me, Billy, or shall I call someone else to hold Burt still?"

"No," Billy said, showing true grit, "I'll hold him!"

Billy took a grip on Burt, and I pushed the hook all the way through the frog's lip, snipping the barbed point off and then easing it out. "There we go, Billy. That should do it. Now let's put him back in the sack. You can let him go in the same spot where you caught him."

Clearly relieved after so much tension, Billy slipped Burt into his paper bag and patted the side of the sack. Smiling happily, he and his mom departed. But the memory lingered on.

All those freckles!

I remembered myself at about Billy's age. I was a terror to frogs. That was back in 1960 before the environmental movement started. Like most of my childhood friends, I didn't appreciate living creatures in the proper reference frame. The good Lord only knows how many frogs I killed. Perhaps our wildlife program would help to teach youngsters of the north woods what I hadn't known when I was a boy like Billy.

Yes, I thought, Billy was a good kid, and I was glad I'd been able to help him. Freeing Burt from the fishhook didn't exactly even my score with the frog world. But it was a beginning. . . .

Though Burt was my· first and last frog to date, I treated some of his cold-blooded relatives. In fact, I averaged two or three turtles each year. Invariably the cause of injury was the same: turtles run over by automobiles. In these cases there wasn't anything I could do. Usually the turtles were dead on arrival. Just the same, I acquired a couple of textbooks on the creatures in case a day came when I could help. The turtle that arrived during July 1981 was not one of those cases.

"What happened?" I asked the woman and teenage boy in the exam room. "Did you accidentally run over the turtle?"

The mother and son had wrapped the turtle in a beach towel,

and I drew the covering aside for a closer look. The shell was cracked in two places, and the pieces were separated widely. Blood oozed from the turtle's nose and mouth. I glanced up at the two wide-eyed onlookers. "Well, I'm sure it wasn't your fault. It's too late to save it, though. The turtle is dead."

"We didn't hit it," the woman volunteered. "The car in front of us did it. The driver swerved over into the other lane, just to hit the turtle!"

"He did," said the boy. "I saw it, too. He did it on purpose. Went way across the center line just to get it."

"Well, there's not much we can do now. I'll bury it. But thank you for trying."

The boy and woman nodded and left, downcast.

I lifted the turtle and took it back to the sink for a closer check. My brother Race was in the treatment room with a hospitalized cat. "Come over here," I said, "and have a look at this turtle."

"What kind is it?" Race took a closer look. "I've never seen one like that before."

The turtle was about ten inches long with black carapace covered with a profusion of tiny, irregularly shaped yellow spots. The head was rather flat, dark on top but with a bright yellow chin and throat.

"Didn't you take a herpetology course a couple of years back?" I asked.

"Yeah," said Race, "but I can't remember every species."

"I'll get the Audubon field guide. Why don't you rinse the blood off it? I'll be right back."

Moments later, I returned with the book, flipping through the pages to the color plate section on turtles. "Here it is, Race. It's a Blanding's turtle."

Race scrutinized the picture. "That's it, all right!"

We began examining the turtle. The first of the two cracks were over the thorax, revealing its insides and the heart. Turtles have a three-chambered heart rather than a four-chambered one

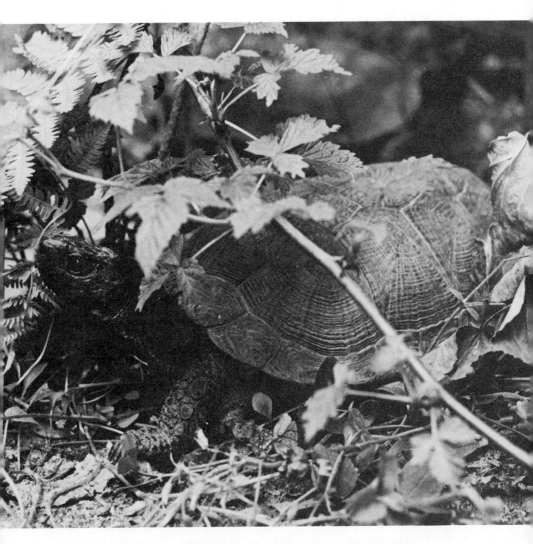

*A box turtle ambles away through the woods
after its cracked shell was repaired.*

like mammals. The ventricle had ruptured. But the two atria appeared intact.

The lungs were crushed completely. But turtles do have an alternate method of respiration for use in crises. They can take in water through the anus and remove oxygen by passing it over primitive gill-like membranes. This backup system was of no use to this turtle now.

The other crack was over the abdominal cavity. Race pulled the shell apart an inch or so, and we peered inside.

"Do you remember your anatomy, Race?"

"Sure." He grabbed an instrument from the drawer and began pointing to the structures inside. "Here's the liver up here, and that's the gallbladder." He moved the pointer slightly. "There's the pancreas and the small and large intestines. Kidneys here. And if you look real close, you can see that clump of dark tissue." He directed the instrument deeper. "Adrenal glands. Ah, and here are the ovaries. Not so much different from the organs of the so-called higher life forms."

The last time I'd seen the internal workings of a turtle had been back at Michigan State in vertebrate physiology class.

Animals were sometimes used in the lab portion of Physiology 565 to emphasize points in the lecture. We had just completed the study of the effect of certain drugs or chemicals on the heart; the lab used turtles to illustrate those effects.

Each pair of students was assigned a turtle. Prior to class the professor had anesthetized all twenty-six of the cold-blooded creatures and hooked them to electrocardiographic monitoring equipment. A section of the shell of each turtle had been removed to enable us to see the heart as well as monitor it.

Our task for the two-hour period was to give different drugs, like epinephrine, the "flight or fight" drugs, into the turtle's bloodstream and watch the changes in the heart's function.

The pathetic part was that everything we "proved" had been known for three decades. It was all very basic, very easy physiology that every student in class knew. For that matter, anyone who could read could have found this information, too.

Now Race placed the turtle in the sink. "Do you want some more info on turtles? My memory's starting to come back now."

"Sure. Why not?"

"Well, one unusual thing is the ribs. They're fused to the underside of the back. And the shoulder and hip joints are inside. Turtles are the only vertebrate with upper limb joints inside the ribs. Think about it.

"Turtles were on earth about two hundred million years ago. Their protective shell is so strong, and their ability to withdraw into it is so successful that they've changed very little. No reason for them to evolve into anything else!"

As I listened to Race talk, something nagged at my mind. "Wait a minute," I said. I hurried back to my office, where I dug out a pamphlet on endangered and threatened Wisconsin species. And there it was: the Blanding's turtle. I dropped the pamphlet and ran back to Race where I shared this information.

Race shook his head in disgust. "Just think. These turtles have been on this planet for two hundred million years. I can't even imagine that amount of time. And now they may disappear."

This turtle had died for no reason that made any sense to me. I looked at the turtle in the sink. More dark red blood leaked from the gaping cracks in the shell. Settling the score for the turtle world would be a long time in coming.

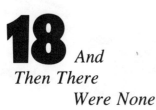 **18** *And Then There Were None*

"Hargus? That's a nice name. It seems to fit him, too," I told Race. We stood looking at a very young great blue heron. "Did you name him?"

"No, Karen did. She thinks every patient must have a name."

"When did it come in?"

"About twenty minutes ago while you were in surgery. I admitted him."

"What's the story?"

"Not much to tell. Two hikers found him beside Bittersweet Lake. He couldn't fly and didn't move. They picked him up and brought him along to us."

The immature bird stood about two feet high. Nearly half that height was in long spindly legs. The beak was six inches long with a very sharp point.

"He looks weak," I said, "but he might peck, if he got the chance. Let's watch it!"

Race held the beak in one hand while we examined the long wings. We discovered that Hargus had a compound fracture of the left radius and ulna. The wound was several days old and filled with maggots. We had our work cut out for us. We spent the next hour removing the maggots one by one.

Our success rate with several-day-old compound fractures in birds wasn't good. But successful healing of the bones was Hargus's only chance. We decided to move ahead with surgery at once. Great Blue herons were on the Wisconsin "watch" list. We didn't want to give up without a fight.

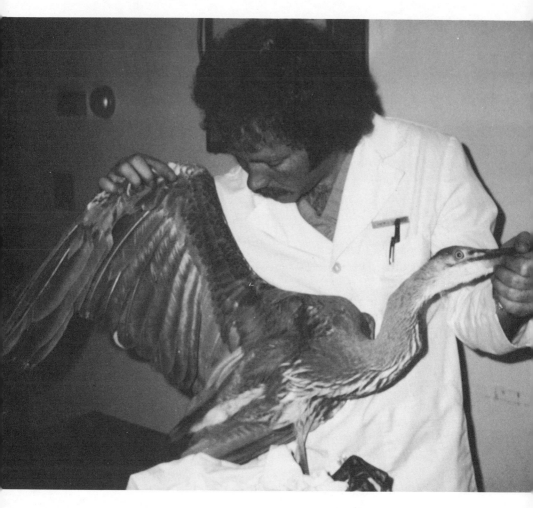

The author examining an injured great blue heron

Race fixed the broken bones, while I monitored the anesthetic. He placed a stainless-steel intramedullary pin through the inside of the ulna to align the broken segments. Then, postoperatively, we applied a splint to the wing and gave the heron antibiotics, disguised in fish, for seven days.

For the next few weeks Hargus lived in a three-foot-wide dog run. The adjacent canine patients didn't seem to disturb him at all. Actually, Hargus seemed to enjoy their company.

Once he'd established his territory, though, he began terrorizing his ward mates. His periodic vocal outbursts scared the dogs half to death. The kennel was Hargus's domain!

All in all, we found the heron's irascibility somewhat humorous, until he stuck his head out and pecked a miniature poodle that happened to walk past the wire front of his run. The peck didn't draw blood, but it must've been painful. The poodle cried like a baby for ten minutes.

"Okay," I said, "you're in trouble, Hargus." I taped cardboard across the front of his run so that he couldn't stick his beak out and cause more damage. But the noise didn't stop. The squawking went unabated.

We kept the kennel doors closed now, but Hargus's periodic squawks could be heard throughout the hospital. Clients made inquiries. What were we harboring? When we explained, nobody minded. It was all okay, but "Boy, what a racket!"

"Kewaaah!" Hargus shrieked.

I was vaccinating George Brooks's dog in the exam room nearest the kennel. George looked up at me, startled. "What in the hell was that?"

"Oh, just our resident blue heron back in the kennel. Weird, huh?"

"*Eerie*'s more like it," said George.

"Kewaaah!" went Hargus.

"What happened to him?" George asked.

"We don't know. He came in a while back with a broken wing."

"He wasn't brought in from Emerson Lake, was he?"

"No, Bittersweet Lake. Why do you ask?"

"Kewaaah!" Hargus squawked.

George shuddered and said, "I live on Emerson, and the guy three houses down from me has been shooting at a blue heron that's been coming to his trout pound."

"What!" I looked at George intently. "Are you sure?"

"Sure, I'm sure. The subject was brought up at a lake owners' association meeting just two nights ago. Several of the property owners were upset when they heard gunshots. We called him and asked him to stop it."

"What did he say?"

"He told us that it was perfectly legal for him to shoot the heron. He claims it was eating the trout he'd stocked in his pond. Anyway, he got a permit from the DNR office to kill it."

My mouth dropped open. "Wait a minute. That's impossible. Blue herons are on the Wisconsin 'watch' list. That means their numbers may be declining. Even the DNR couldn't issue a permit to shoot one . . . could they?" Suddenly I was having doubts. My years of experience with the DNR told me *anything* was possible.

George shrugged. "He showed us his permit."

"George, would you be kind enough to give me this guy's name? I'd like to call him. I won't mention your name at all."

George agreed.

After he departed with his dog, I phoned the alleged heron shooter, Ben Herter. I told him, "I understand you're having a problem with a blue heron in your area. Just called to see if I could help."

"It's no problem of yours," said Herter. "I've got a blue heron that's eating my trout, and I have a solution. I got a permit from the DNR to shoot it. It's perfectly legal."

"Sir," I said, "I think there must be some mistake. Great blue herons are protected, both on a state and federal level. They're even on a special list in our state, demanding our protection."

"That's a mistake," Herter shot back. "I have a permit right here. It's from the local DNR office. If you want to check, call the office."

Obviously Herter had the permit. Since I was making no headway on that front, I tried a different tack. "Are you sure it's the heron that's eating your trout? Herons pretty much stick to the shallows. Trout like deeper water."

"All I know is there aren't many trout in my pond. I stocked it last fall. I've seen the heron. He *must* be eating them."

"Often herons just wade along the shorelines looking for minnows or crayfish. I know you think it's the heron that's eating your trout, but maybe it's not." I was trying to be diplomatic.

"As I said before, this is no concern of yours." Herter hung up.

Now I thought of calling the DNR. But knowing them all too well, I knew it was pointless.

Two weeks later we removed the pin from Hargus's wing. I released him on the southern shore of Lake Tomahawk, watching him leap into the air from the lily pad on which I placed him.

As he flew down the lake, I called after him, "Stay away from trout ponds, Hargus!"

19
Snowflake

I was talking on the telephone with Karl Olson, a good fishing buddy who worked in the nuclear research department of Berkeley Labs, an institution affiliated with the University of California.

"How are things in the north woods?" he asked.

"Great," I replied. "And how are things in California?" Although we lived far from each other, Karl and I maintained regular, if infrequent, contact.

Ten minutes into the conversation, Karl arrived at his reason for telephoning on this August evening. "Listen, Ror, I have a couple of weeks off in September. I'm thinking of going to Alaska fishing and backpacking. Want to come with me?"

"Alaska!" I exclaimed. What an idea! I'd been thinking of taking some time off and going fishing, but I'd planned to do my fishing in my own neck of the woods.

"That's right," Karl went on. "With the deregulation, the air fares are a bargain. I have a friend living on Kenai Peninsula, so it won't cost much once we get there."

I thought of these last two years I'd spent reading *Alaska* magazine. I was attracted to the country, intrigued by its wilderness. "It sounds great," I admitted. "Marty and Race can hold down the fort." Quickly I was talking myself into making the trip. "And, hey, I'm sure Linda wouldn't mind." There was only one possible problem. "Race, my brother, has to return to vet school on September twenty-eighth. Would we be back by then?"

Karl did a quick rundown of the trip. "We'll leave on the

eighth and return on the twenty-fourth. The timing is perfect for you!''

Karl was absolutely right. Meanwhile, I could justify taking some time off. I hadn't had a real vacation in nearly four years. "Okay," I decided, "I'll go. Why don't you send me your flight plans, and I'll hook up with you in Seattle. We can go on from there together. You'd better send me a list of things I'll need in Alaska, though. I haven't done much backpacking.''

On August 23 I sat down to make my plans. My itinerary had me leaving Wisconsin at 6:02 A.M., September 8, flight 197 from Central Wisconsin Airport, about ninety-five miles from my home in Minocqua. By September 7, I had my gear laid out and ready to pack. I was scheduled to go off duty at 5:30 P.M., and I didn't have to leave for the airport until 4:00 A.M. Everything was going smoothly. I would even have time for a pleasant dinner with my family.

Dinner came and went, a festive occasion—a kind of going-away party for dear old dad. Then the phone rang.

I pushed myself away from the table, stuffed with Linda's good cooking, saying, "Probably someone wanting to say good-bye."

It was Race.

"What's up, pal?" I asked him.

"Marty and I are at the Dairymen's Country Club," Race said, "and we wondered if you could meet us up here and help us look for an injured deer."

Knowing Race, I sensed this was another of his pranks. "Oh, sure, Race," I said. "And how about you and Marty meeting me on Trout Lake to look for an injured fish?"

Race laughed. "No, Rory, I'm serious. We need help.''

Although I now knew Race wasn't joking, I protested, "It's dark outside. How are you going to find an injured deer? Is it close to the road or something?"

Race got down to brass tacks. He and Marty had been summoned out to the Dairymen's Club, a private ten-thousand-acre retreat, to investigate a possibly injured deer named Snowflake, a rare albino doe. After six years of living on the private wildlife refuge, Snowflake had become the lodge owners' favorite. Since hunting was prohibited, some of the wild animals, especially the deer, had little fear of man. Though they were not confined, the deer had become quite friendly. Snowflake was one of several deer that were tame enough to be hand-fed. Evidently she had been hit by a car earlier that day on one of the few roads leading to the secluded cabins. She had disappeared into the woods, later wandering close to the main lodge, where caretakers had observed a dangling rear leg. Alarmed, they had telephoned our hospital for help.

When Race and Marty had arrived at the Dairymen's Club, twenty-five miles north of Minocqua, Snowflake stood nervously on the edge of the lawn near the lodge. One look confirmed the caretakers' suspicions. Snowflake could put no weight on the injured leg; with each step it swayed back and forth, leaving the trained observer no doubt that she had a broken bone.

The difficult decision was what to do about it. Both of them had worked on enough deer to know that external casts and splints on an adult deer were a waste of time. The animals wouldn't tolerate any device fastened to the outside of a leg, no matter how securely it was placed.

Race and Marty had decided on the only feasible course of action: repairing the broken bone by implanting a rigid internal support. In the case of an adult deer, this meant using a stainless steel plate—a bone plate. This could be screwed directly into the bone, accomplishing solid reduction of the fracture and eliminating the need for support outside the leg.

Race and Marty had decided to repair the bone on the spot and as soon as possible. With each passing hour the dangling leg was becoming more and more bruised and swollen. They had driven back to the animal hospital to secure all the items needed for out-clinic surgery: full surgery pack, all the bone equipment, the inhalation anesthetic machine, and all ancillary supplies. In other words, they had packed Marty's truck with five thousand dollars' worth of medical equipment.

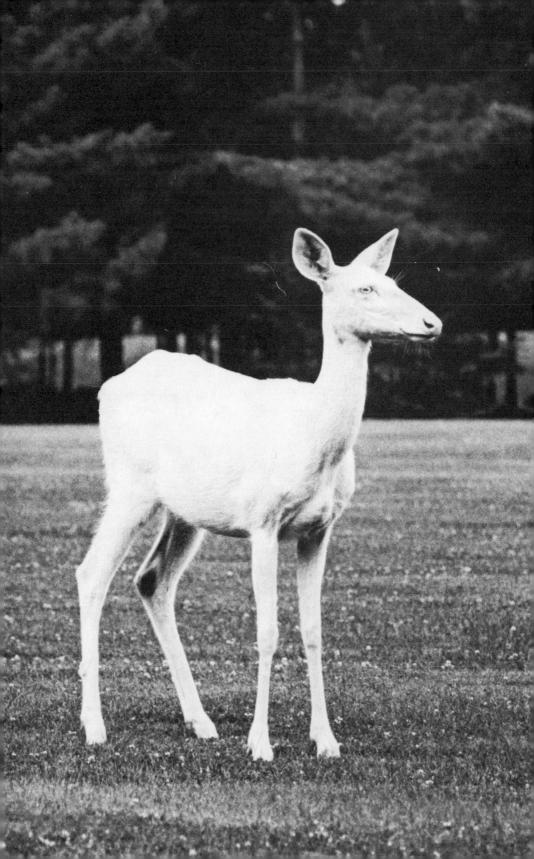

They had arrived back at the Dairymen's Club shortly after dark. The first task—anesthetizing Snowflake—proved more difficult than they had expected. The car accident, along with the extra attention, had made her apprehensive and wild. We didn't own a tranquilizer gun, and the doe didn't want to hold still while they injected the anesthetic. Consequently a half-hour chase had followed.

Once they caught the patient, Marty managed to get only a partial dose of anesthetic into Snowflake. The prick of the needle had alarmed her, and the deer had bolted into the nearby woods.

"How about it?" ended Race. "We need your help!"

Despite my pending departure for Alaska, Race's story got to me. The whole adventure seemed unbelievable, almost comical, and definitely an event not to miss. We had never done surgery outside the clinic before!

As I turned off County Trunk B toward the entrance to the private club, I marveled at the unique setting. The owners of the Dairymen's Club had purchased the acreage, including seven lakes, sixty years before and had seen to it that the area remained untouched.

A mile from the lodge a huge black bear and two cubs lumbered across the road, heading north toward Wolf Lake. They disappeared into the virgin pines, all of which had to be over a century old.

At last, among the massive trunks of the pine trees, the glow of a yard light appeared. I must be nearing the lodge. I passed several rustic log cabins, used by club members for summer outings, and proceeded toward the light.

Near the lodge itself was Marty's green Ford truck, parked beside a small square shed. The passenger door of the truck was open, evidence of Race's hurried departure. As my car lights

Snowflake, the albino deer

illuminated the truck, two shining eyes reflected from the front seat.

I watched closely as a hungry raccoon scurried from the truck carrying in its mouth a lunch bag, no doubt a remnant of one of Marty's fishing excursions. Then a blond woman came out of the lighted shed. She rushed to meet me as I braked to a halt, calling to me, "Hi, Dr. Foster. I'm Bonnie, one of the caretakers. I'm trying to get this shed ready for surgery. The guys are all over the woods looking for Snowflake." She pointed to the dark forest behind her, handing me a flashlight as I stepped out to meet her. "Here. Take this and help, if you like."

Armed with a five-cell flashlight, I stood behind the shed for a few minutes, watching and listening intently. A coyote yapped; otherwise, silence prevailed. Then I saw a flickering of light in the woods. I turned my flashlight in that direction and headed out. Three hundred yards into the trees I came upon Race.

"We haven't found her yet," Race said. "But a few minutes ago we heard something crash through the leaves over there." He pointed his flashlight. "We're trying to comb this general area."

I was about to open my mouth to reply, when Marty yelled, "Hey, I found her. I found her!"

We began running toward Marty's voice. As we came upon him, we saw that he was sitting awkwardly on the 150-pound albino doe. She struggled in vain, but with the sedation she didn't have enough energy to free herself from Marty.

Marty was soaked in perspiration. "Hurry," he said. "Give her another injection." He handed me a syringe.

I fumbled with the needle cap. Finally, I got my act together and injected anesthetic into Snowflake's flank. The higher dosage caused her to fall into a deep sleep within a minute or two.

The three of us carried her to a small road Marty had discovered a short distance away. Race hurried back to the lodge and brought around my four-wheel-drive Bronco to transport the

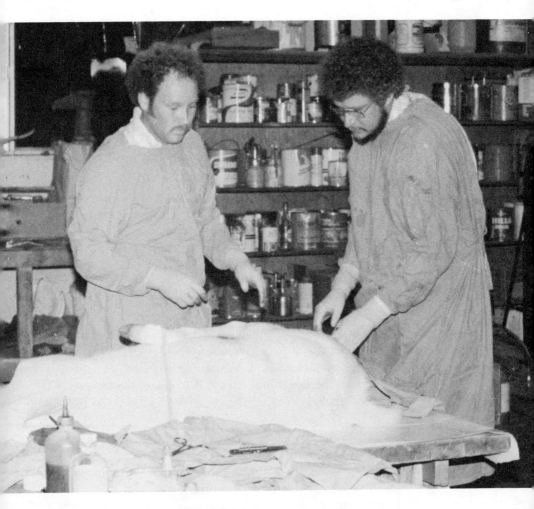

*The author (left) and Dr. Smith, donned in
surgical garb, proceed with surgery on Snowflake.
The modern technique used for fracture repair
stands in sharp contrast to the antiquated shed
in which the surgery was performed.*

doe to the shed, which he and Marty had turned into a makeshift surgery room.

With Bonnie's help we prepared for surgery. Someone had found a large slab of half-inch-thick plywood and had placed it across two ancient sawhorses; this would serve as a surgery table. We placed the doe on the table and immediately began an intravenous solution, the liter bottle hanging from a wooden stepladder. Above the surgical table hung an antiquated Coca-Cola mirror; despite the years of dust and fading, the Coca-Cola girl of a bygone era smiled energetically from an old wooden frame. All around us, pushed aside for the time being, was the litter of the shed: an orange Toro tractor, several empty barrels, a rusty double-bladed ax with a cracked handle, a set of deer antlers mounted on a tarnished plaque bearing the trophy's date—1952. This wasn't the perfect setting for surgery, but it would do in an emergency such as this.

Since the injectable anesthetic wasn't intended for a lengthy surgical procedure, we passed an endotracheal tube down the doe's trachea to administer the inhalation anesthetic. This would keep the doe under for as long as necessary.

Passing a trach tube in most animals is fairly easy. But due to the anatomy of the doe's oral cavity, it's impossible to open the mouth wide enough to see the trachea. We had to insert the tube "by feel."

Race pulled on Snowflake's moist pink tongue as I felt in the back of her narrow mouth for the trachea. I couldn't locate it at first, and my rigorous probing aroused Snowflake. Soft brown eyes blinked slowly; she swallowed several times.

"Hurry," Race said. "She's waking up."

"I'm trying. I'm trying. There. I think I can feel it." I slipped the tube down. As I did so, Snowflake clamped her mouth shut tightly.

"Yikes!" I yelled, jerking my hand from her mouth. I gasped and looked at my throbbing index finger. Her closing molars had bruised and lacerated the middle finger joint and my own red blood dripped to the cement floor. "Marty! Turn the anesthetic all the way up!"

Marty cranked the lever on the machine to full open.

While we waited for Snowflake to settle down, I bandaged my finger. Finally, my wound attended to and Snowflake asleep again, we proceeded.

Palpation of her injured hind limb revealed a midshaft fracture of the tibia, the bone between the knee to the hock. We clipped the short white hair from the sleek leg and scrubbed the area with Betadine surgical scrub for sterile surgery. Now Marty and I donned full surgery gowns while Race tended to the anesthetic and intravenous fluids. Soon we were at work.

We applied a dynamic compression bone plate—actually intended for human use—to the side of the tibia. The eight-inch stainless-steel plate spanned the fracture site. We anchored it above and below by placing three screws through the plate into the bone. The thick, three-quarter-inch-wide plate, once secured, was stronger than the original bone. This eliminated the need for any other support. The two broken ends of the bone, thus held in apposition, should heal nicely, and the plate could stay on forever. The surgery was long and tiresome. Two whole hours passed before we stepped back from the makeshift surgical table.

Feeling good about what we had done here tonight, we lifted Snowflake from the table and carried her to a grassy knoll behind the shed to recover. While we stood there, waiting for her to exhibit some signs of consciousness, I realized how late it was.

"Oh, my God," I said, "I haven't packed, and I've gotta leave in two hours! Stick with it!" I raced for the Bronco, made it home in record time, and ran into the house.

I packed quickly, took a brief shower, grabbed a bit of breakfast, kissed everyone good-bye, promising to have a good time, and broke another record driving to the airport.

As the plane flew west, I slept over Minnesota, South Dakota, Montana, Idaho, and Washington, exhausted. In Seattle, the stewardess awakened me.

Since I had a few minutes before Karl's flight arrived, I telephoned Marty at the clinic to inquire about Snowflake.

"She came out of the anesthetic in good shape," Marty told me. "Bonnie called me about midmorning and said Snowflake was nibbling grass."

Elated, I hung up the phone, reflecting on the events of the night before—the difficult capture and the challenge of complicated surgery. Snowflake just might be the only wild deer anywhere with a bone plate in her leg. Certainly she was an albino deer of distinction!

Feeling good, I stepped out of the telephone booth, confident I had earned my vacation. Then I spotted Karl coming toward me. It was time to go fishing.

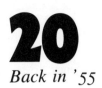

Back in '55

I grew up in the small southern Michigan community of Allegan, not far from Lake Michigan. The town was bordered on three sides by farmland and on the fourth by the Allegan State Forest. The forest was the only wild area in that otherwise agricultural region, and it offered an array of outdoor activities: hiking, camping, fishing, hunting, and trapping.

My father knew the forest as well as anyone did. He hunted there, but he was best at trapping fox. He loved to tell Race and me about his trapping days in the forest, and he had one story that we must've heard a hundred times during our growing-up years.

The year of the story was 1955. Always my father began his favorite tale the same way: "Back in 'fifty-five . . ." The beginning was so predictable that Race and I referred to it as the "Back in 'fifty-five" story.

Our dad had been scouting in the forest in preparation for the trapping season, and he stopped at the ranger station to discuss the fox-trapping prospects. By sheer luck, the head game biologist for the district happened to be at the ranger station that day.

"I'm Clayton Foster," Dad said when he entered the station. "I'm thinking of doing some red fox trapping around here. I'm wondering if there's many around this year."

The biologist stepped forward and said, "Well, Mr. Foster, there are no fox around here to trap. I've checked the area myself and haven't seen so much as a track. There's just no fox around this year."

Dad thanked the man and departed. But being the skeptic he was, especially of schooled game biologists, he decided to check for himself.

The forest was scattered with small sand dunes, so he drove down the gravel road apiece, then hiked a short distance into the forest in search of fox tracks. Sure enough, Dad found a sand dune loaded with fox prints.

Dad ended up having his most successful year trapping foxes, and he trapped most of them within a five-mile radius of the ranger station.

Dad got great mileage from that story. He loved to tell it to his trapping buddies, too. Meanwhile, he became more skeptical of the local conservation department. "If they don't know what a fox track looks like," he said, laughing, "then what *do* they know?"

I hadn't thought of that story in almost ten years, until a green International Scout with "University of Wisconsin" stamped on its doors backed right up to the entrance of the hospital one morning. What caught our attention was not so much the fact that the university vehicle had come so far up into the woods as it was the huge circular antenna mounted on the Scout's roof. The apparatus was two feet high and two feet in diameter.

"What's that thing on top?" I asked Marty as we looked through the glass doors at the Scout.

"Looks like a tracking device. We used those in the army."

"What would the university be tracking up here?"

"Beats me," said Marty. Then he grinned. "Maybe someone's spotted Bigfoot. Who knows?"

Two men in their mid-twenties climbed from the Scout and opened up its back. Inside was a full-grown coyote stretched out on a piece of plywood.

"Guess we better see what goes on," I said.

"Yeah, I think I saw the coyote breathing."

We stepped outside. Yes, the coyote was alive.

"What's the problem?" I asked.

"She's been heavily drugged so we could get her here," one of the young men in blue jeans explained.

"We brought her in so you could check her leg," the other fellow said.

I looked at the coyote closely. The rear legs appeared to be okay, but there was an obvious swelling high on the right paw. "What happened to her?"

"She was caught in a trap by that foot there," said the first fellow. "We gave her a shot of anesthetic and got her out. We need it checked."

Marty, silent until now, said, "I must have missed something here. Why was she trapped and why do you want the wound checked? From the Scout it's obvious you guys are from the university. Are you doing some sort of research?"

"Sorry," said the second guy. "I guess I should explain. I'm Mike Sutton, and this is Charlie Whittier. We're graduate students at the university. We're working on our master's degrees in wildlife management. We're trying to determine the home range of the coyote. How much territory a coyote will cover in a day or a week. Stuff like that. You know, for management purposes in the future. We trap coyotes and place radio transmitters on their collars. Then we monitor their movements with the telemetry equipment on the Scout."

"So that's what the antenna's for," Marty said.

"Yep," said Mike. "It's for tracking coyotes."

"Well, let's take the coyote inside, Rory, and X-ray the paw. Okay?"

I nodded, and the two students lifted the large female coyote from the Scout.

Mike was the typical clean-cut college student. He had short blond hair under a red and white Badgers cap. He seemed well mannered and easygoing.

His companion, Charlie, was more reserved. He reminded me of a merit scholar with his short curly hair and horn-rimmed glasses.

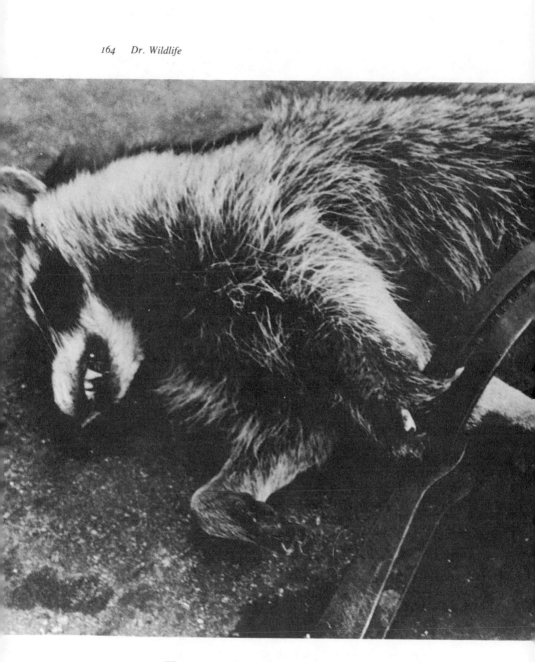

There must be a better answer than traps.

I held the double doors open, and they carried the coyote into the hospital. Marty directed them to the radiology room, where he took two separate X-rays of the paw, one from the front and one from the side. Then I developed the radiographs.

I entered the small darkroom and closed the door behind me. The only light was the faint orange glow from the X-ray light mounted at eye level on the wall beside the developing tank. I removed the exposed films from the two cassettes and clipped them onto the hangers for insertion into the tank. Next I placed fresh film in the cassettes for future use.

Ordinarily I would have picked up the timer and left the room for the five minutes required to develop the X-rays. But the darkroom seemed peaceful to me today, and I stayed an extra few moments. I was thinking of those two guys and their research.

What good would it do to monitor a coyote to determine its home range, if its foot was broken or bruised? Since coyotes don't run in packs, an injured coyote wasn't going to range far. Since the research project didn't make sense to me, I decided to ask the scholar a few questions.

I opened the door and squinted into the brighter light of the room. Marty had anticipated my question. "In your research," he was saying, "how do you take into account the fact that the coyotes are injured? Doesn't that affect their range?"

"Oh," said Charlie, "we don't put transmitters on the ones with fractures. For example, if she has a broken paw, we won't use her." He nodded to the coyote lying on the floor beside the X-ray table.

Now here was a tempting conversation. I stepped out and said, "But sometimes the foot can be severely damaged without broken bones. Last year I treated a Labrador retriever that was caught in a trap. The dog had no broken bones. The foot appeared normal for two days. Then the skin sloughed off, and the toes died. We ended up amputating the paw!"

Charlie shrugged and looked away. "Well, we don't have

any other way to catch coyotes. They're too smart to walk into live traps."

"That doesn't make your method scientifically justifiable, though," I challenged, "even if it is the only way!"

The timer went off, and I hurried to attend to the X-rays. But while I was inside the darkroom I could still hear the conversation. As I rinsed the X-rays and placed them in the fixative for several minutes prior to reading, I heard Marty saying, "You know, Dr. Foster is right. We get ten or fifteen trap injuries each year. It's not always easy to determine the extent of the damage. Even if the bones are all right, the tendons, nerves, or blood vessels can be crushed beyond repair. You can't always tell right away about those things. Those injuries could take weeks or even months to heal, and as Dr. Foster told you, they may not heal at all."

I opened the door, bringing the X-rays with me, and placed them on the viewer. Two broken bones. Not just hairline fractures. The bones were snapped apart!

Since the bones would likely heal on their own, Mike and Charlie picked up their still sedated coyote and went their way.

When the door had closed behind them, I turned to Marty and said, "I know you think I come down too hard on the DNR and the wildlife management people, but you know damn well the data they're collecting are worthless."

"Those guys aren't managers yet," said Marty. "Remember, they're just students!"

"Stuff and nonsense," I fumed. "They'll probably publish their findings in some wildlife management journal, after drawing all kinds of erroneous conclusions. Anyway, I'm sure they're working in cooperation with the DNR. This isn't even trapping season, you know."

"You're right," Marty admitted. "Their research project is stupid. The coyotes probably don't like it either. That coyote could lose her foot."

I was astounded. "You mean you *agree* with me?"

"Only if you'll buy lunch, Foster."

I hesitated. "One more thing, Marty. I wonder if those guys know what a fox track looks like."

Marty stepped back. "A fox track? What's that got to do with it, Foster?"

Rather than go into my father's favorite story, I said, "Come on. Lunch is on me."

Race arrived in early November from Michigan State. The two of us and my father spent a weekend fishing for muskie.

We were out on Star Lake casting for the elusive muskie when I told Race and my father about the coyote incident. Of course, I ended up delivering a tirade against research that hurts animals and proves nothing. "And these guys could be professional wildlife managers someday!"

My father turned from his position in the bow of the boat where he'd been fishing intently. "That reminds me of another story," he began. "Did I ever tell you boys about my fox-trapping days and the time I talked to the game manager in Allegan?"

Race and I glanced at each other grinning. Then Race reached down to the six-pack of beer. He handed me one and took one for himself.

"No, Dad," I said. "Can't say I ever heard that one."

"Me either," said Race, warming to the story with a sip of his beer. "Tell us."

Snow began to fall, wet snow, coming down fast. Already yesterday's snow was disappearing under a new white blanket, beautiful to the eye.

I studied my father. His cheeks were red from the rising wind that bit into the flesh, and the fresh wet snow clung to his handlebar mustache. He wasn't cold, though. His eyes were sparkling with the delight of remembrances long past.

"Well, boys," he said, "let's see now. If I remember correctly, it was back in 'fifty-five . . ."

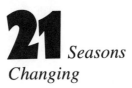**21** *Seasons Changing*

I thought the spring of 1982 would never arrive. But that's how it always is after a long, bitter north woods winter.

As if to prove we're not in control of such matters, winter blasts our country sometimes as late as May with several inches of snow. Never mind the calendar, which promises spring on March 20. Northern Wisconsin is a whole different ball game.

Bird-watchers mark the seasonal change by the first sight of a loon or a robin. Canoeing enthusiasts recognize spring when the Tomahawk River opens and becomes navigable. Fishermen hail winter's exit with the opening day of fishing, the first Saturday in May. But for me, a veterinarian interested in wildlife, winter isn't officially gone until someone brings me the first newborn wild patient.

In 1982, this event occurred on a cold and dreary day— May 17, to be exact, at 6:18 in the evening.

I was in the lab finishing up some blood tests, when Karen came in. "Dr. Foster," she said, "there's a couple in the first exam room with an injured rabbit. It's Jim and Beverly Kline. You remember them. They have two Irish setters, Max and Sampson, and a cat, Calypso."

"Sure," I said, smiling in recollection. They'd been bringing their animals to me for treatment since I opened the hospital in 1976. Beverly was very nice, but her husband Jim was something of a pain in the neck. He had bred and raised Irish setters, and he thought he knew more than any veterinarian about them. "How could I forget!" I laughed. "What's Jim's problem *now?*"

"Well," said Karen, "he's at it again. He and his wife are arguing about this rabbit. I don't think he wanted to bring it in. But his wife insisted."

"Can the rabbit wait a second? I need to finish this blood glucose check on the diabetic dog."

"That's okay," Karen said. "The rabbit isn't bleeding. I'll tell them it'll be a few minutes."

Karen had hardly delivered the news when Jim's and Beverly's voices rose to new heights in argument. They could be heard all over the hospital. As I did my blood work, I listened in.

"I don't care what you say," Jim was saying, "this is a waste of time! What sense does it make to try to save one rabbit when there's hundreds of them out there!" Jim was really pouring it on, fire and brimstone at its best.

"Jim, don't get so upset. The lawn mower killed the other three in the nest. The least we can do is try and help this one. Maybe Dr. Foster can fix him."

"Ridiculous!" snapped Jim. "We drove six miles in here. Now I've missed the evening news. We gotta go all the way back just for this damn bunny!"

I smiled to myself. I couldn't imagine Jim using the word "bunny." There was something wonderfully incongruous about that remark.

"Anyway," Jim sailed on, in fine form, "it'll probably die. If you hadn't been home, I'd've done the proper thing—put it out of its misery. What's the difference? It's only a bunny rabbit!"

There it was again—bunny. I stifled my roar of laughter.

"I don't care!" Beverly yelled back at him. "The poor little thing deserves a chance. It's not his fault you mowed over his nest."

"Oh, Bev!" groaned Jim. "This is nature's way that some animals die. You've seen too many Bambi movies. You just don't understand. It's the way of the wild!"

"Oh, I see," Beverly said, "you figure your lawn mower is an instrument of nature! Baloney! If one of us doesn't understand, it's not me, it's you!"

"Oh, for Christ's sake, here we go again with that crap!

Look, Beverly. Even if the rabbit gets better, he'll probably be eaten by something in the woods. Some coyote will get him. Bringing him here is futile. He's still going to die. Jesus!''

"Well, at least it won't be you and your lawn mower that did him in. He deserves a chance. Anyway, Dr. Foster will work on him for free. It's not going to cost you a penny. You sound as if you're going to have to pay for it.''

"I can see helping eagles and loons and such, but a rabbit? Really, Beverly, get a grip on yourself. Foster's got better things to do.''

"Like what?'' Beverly shot back. "Play golf like you! Maybe he thinks things like that are a waste of time. Think about that. Anyway, it won't be your time or money being spent. Why should you care?''

"If you ask me,'' Jim shouted, "Dr. Foster is an eccentric if he wastes his time on rabbits. It's not just me saying this. Plenty of other people are saying it, too. He wastes his time on all kinds of birds and animals.''

The buzzer sounded on the blood chemistry machine to signal the end of the test. I recorded the results and marched to the exam room. I threw open the door and restrained myself. It wasn't easy, but I greeted him as if I'd heard nothing. "What do we have in the box?'' I asked.

Beverly pulled herself together and in a soft, sweet voice said, "There's a newborn bunny in here.'' She set the box on the exam table. "Jim was mowing the lawn and went over its nest. Three of the rabbits were killed. But this one's alive. I think the blade knicked its side, but I do hope it'll be okay.''

Jim didn't say a word; he just glared at his wife and me, sighing in disgust.

"Okay,'' I said. "Thanks for bringing him in. You can leave him with me, and I'll look after him.'' I hoped they would depart; I had no desire to get into a heated debate with either of them with regard to the future of the patient. I ushered them from the room, thanking them for bringing the rabbit along to me.

With the Klines out of my hair, I opened the box, reached

in, and gently lifted the tiny frightened creature to examine its injury. The little rabbit was only about three and a half inches long. Its back was covered with very short soft brown hair, but the coat on its underside was downy white. His tiny pink nose and whiskers wiggled when I placed him on the table.

On the rabbit's left side, beneath the last rib was a neat, orderly incision about one inch in length. Evidently this is where the mower blade had hit. Several loops of small pink intestine were visible through the newly created window. Bits of hair, green grass, and dirt had entered the abdomen. Despite the injury, the bunny sat stoically on the table while I contemplated his fate.

As had happened hundreds of times in the past five years, I had to make a decision about a wild animal's life. Often there was no dilemma or second thought. Certainly I'd never hesitated to treat an eagle or an osprey. Nor did loons or blue herons leave much room for contemplation. But maybe Jim Kline was right about this newborn rabbit. There were hundreds, thousands, maybe millions of exact replicas of this patient out in the wild. The life of this one tiny creature was unimportant to the overall rabbit population. Everyone knew that.

I stood over the frightened little rabbit and began to list mentally all the arguments in favor of humane euthanasia.

Not only was its life unimportant to the rabbit population, but to proceed with treatment would mean keeping Karen another forty-five minutes at least, and it was already nearly seven. Gentle restraint would be required while I shaved the fur from around the wound. Then a thorough cleaning would be necessary to remove the contamination. Next, proper treatment would necessitate using a local anesthetic followed by small, tediously

This baby owl was rendered homeless after an unsuspecting logger chopped down the tree where the owl family was living.

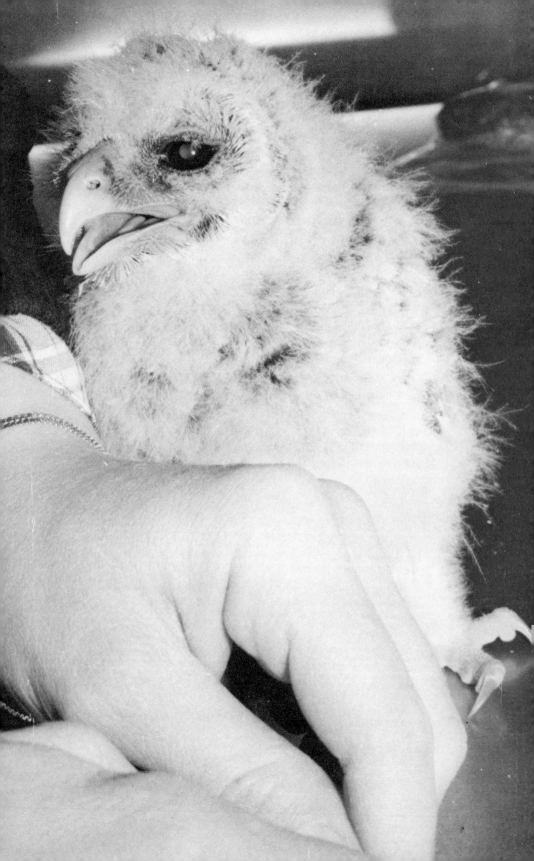

placed sutures to close the wound. Assuming the patient made it through all that, I would have to transport it home for the night and keep it on a heating pad. Either Linda or I would have to get up at least twice during the night to check on it, give it milk with an eyedropper, and administer antibiotics. It did seem like a lot to do for a rabbit.

Even if I stayed and attempted treatment, past experience told me there was only a 50 percent chance of saving the rabbit. And I knew Jim was right about something else: I could spend hours on this creature, and shortly after I released him he could die of something else. There was no question about that; he might be caught by an owl or fox, or get hit by a car.

So in light of all the facts—that this individual was not important in the scheme of things, that it really didn't have a good chance of making it anyway, that it would require hours of nursing care at the end of what had already been a twelve-hour day—I did what I had to do.

Decisions between my heart and my head have never been easy for me.

I arrived home late that night, but Linda didn't mind at all. She even volunteered to get up during the night to help feed the new patient.

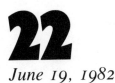

22

June 19, 1982

I awakened with a kink in my neck and a dull ache in my back where I had rested against the pine tree. I checked my watch: 3:30 A.M. My God, I thought, we must've dozed off.

I glanced over at Linda beside me. She was sound asleep, and so was the fawn in her lap.

"Linda," I whispered softly, "wake up, honey. It's three-thirty."

Linda's eyes fought sleep and finally won. "Did you say three-thirty?" she murmured.

"Come on. Let's put the fawn over there on the straw."

We carried the fawn over to the corner of the courtyard where we placed it on the thick mat of straw. Then Linda stroked its head as if it were a small child, and in seconds the fawn was settled in for what remained of the night.

"I wonder if Ali and Mikie are all right," Linda said, her face filled with concern.

"Ah, they've probably been asleep for hours," I consoled her. "Anyway, they've spent the night with your sister before. They're okay. Probably had a ball playing with your sister's kids. Anyway, let's pick them up early. They can come to the opening with us. Ali will want to see the new fawn."

We took our departure from the courtyard through the door into the wildlife hospital. Lights burned there from the activity earlier preparatory to the grand opening, now only five hours away.

Silence was everywhere beneath the bright lights. The wildlife patients were over on the other side, waiting until the opening, when they would be transferred to their new quarters.

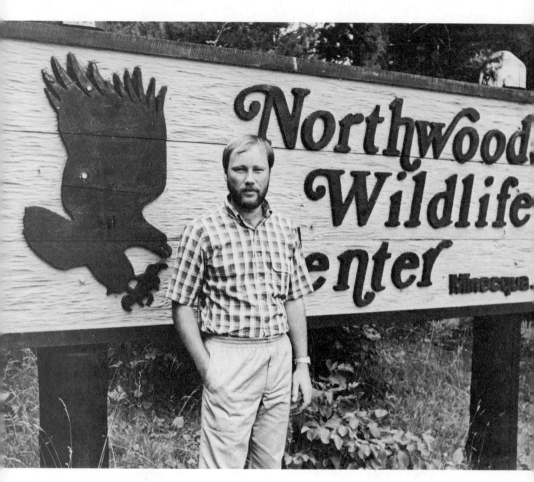

*The author stands beside the sign commemorating
the official opening of the Northwoods Wildlife Center,
Minocqua, Wisconsin.*

"Linda," I murmured, "I feel like walking around in here for a last look. It'll never be this quiet again."

Linda understood. She grabbed my hand, and together we walked through the student apartment, a room conceived to make use of the educational potential of the center. A university student, veterinary or otherwise, could stay here and study aspects of wildlife.

"I wish," I said to Linda, "that I'd had a place like this when I was in school."

The treatment room, adjacent to the student apartment, was our next stop. Cabinets filled with medical supplies lined a wall. A tall brown refrigerator towered in a corner. I opened the refrigerator, smiling. It contained food for the patients, stacks of frozen smelt for the fish eaters, packages of meat scraps supplied free by a local restaurant for the others.

"Water Birds" was printed on the door leading into the next room. The American bittern and blue heron we were treating would be transferred here soon; the deep water trough along the wall would be an ideal place for injured loons and ducks.

Linda and I retraced our steps through the treatment area. The flight room was next.

The flight room was large, with a water bath built into the floor. Birds of prey would be rehabilitated here.

Mindlessly I said, "We have three flight cages outside."

"I know." Linda laughed softly.

I paused and looked at her, my beautiful wife. I kissed her full on the lips. Linda was as much a part of this as I was.

Behind the flight room was another smaller room with cages; they could house just about any type of patient, mammals or birds not ready for the flight room. Any wild creature would be safe in here.

The large reception room could double as a conference or educational room for slide presentations and such. The cabinets on one wall were half filled with books on wildlife. It would take a while to fill the shelves, but we would do it.

As I stepped behind the yellow counter to turn off the light, I noticed the stack of cards bearing the new eagle print by Lee LaBlanc, the Northwoods Wildlife Center's 1982 Artist of the Year. Another stack of *Loons at Dusk,* a picture done by Art Long, our 1981 Artist of the Year, was also there. A box of new brochures describing our project occupied one corner of the room; we hoped to acquire new members at the grand opening.

The new telephone, installed only a week earlier, sat next to the electric typewriter Marty and I had donated to the center. Next to the phone was a small pile of messages from the day before. I leaned closer. On top was a note in Linda's handwriting. I smiled across the counter at her. "Did I have any calls or messages today?"

"Yes, but when that fawn came in, I forgot about everything else." She reached over and picked up the pink slips of paper. "Oh, yes. A man named Tom Beamer called. Said to tell you he'd be here for the opening. Do you know him?"

I laughed in recollection. "I sure do. He was in that day we had the porcupine. Remember?"

Linda smiled. "I remember now."

I pulled out the desk chair and sat down. "What else?"

"Race called and said he's going to drive all night from Michigan State to get here for the opening. He said to tell you his final exams went well. Sounded really fired up!"

"Probably because it's starting to sink in that he's nearly done with school. One more year. Eight years." I shook my head, thinking back briefly to my own days as a veterinary student. "That's a long time."

"Someone from the Dairymen's Club called today," Linda went on. "I'm supposed to tell you, Marty, and Race that Snowflake, the albino deer, had twins this week!"

"Hey, that's great! I'll be sure and tell 'em."

"There's a letter here that I didn't open. It's addressed to you."

"Open it," I said. "Who's it from?"

"Well . . ." She hesitated. "I can't pronounce the name of the town, but it's from a veterinarian in Oregon."

"Oregon?" I didn't know any vets in Oregon.

"Maybe you ought to open this yourself." Linda handed the letter over the counter to me.

With one glance, I was floored. The letter was addressed to Dr. Wildlife, Minocqua, Wisconsin!

Very carefully I opened the letter, which had arrived at my doorstep in spite of its rather inadequate address. I scanned the pages. The vet had a cousin in Wisconsin who had sent him a newspaper article about the opening of the wildlife hospital. In his practice in Oregon, he worked on farm animals and some small animals, but always he'd wanted to work with wildlife. Now he was thinking of starting such a project himself. He was interested in hearing about the kinds of problems I'd encountered, and he wished me the best of luck in the future.

"Well?" said Linda.

I handed the letter to her, surprised and happy. What a nice letter! He had more than likely misplaced the article and forgotten my name, so he had taken a chance on the U.S. Mail, hoping that the letter would arrive at its destination.

After Linda read the letter, she looked up at me slowly and said finally, "What are you going to tell him?"

I leaned forward in my chair not sure how to answer.

"Well," said Linda after a long silence, "what are you going to tell him?"

"I heard you the first time," I said, breaking into laughter. "I guess I'm just going to have to tell him the truth!"

I stood up and grabbed Linda's hand. "Come on. In five hours we gotta be back here."

"Let's check on the fawn one more time."

"Okay, one last time."

We went back to the courtyard to stand looking down on the fawn. "Isn't she beautiful?" Linda said.

"Yes. And she's doing just fine, thanks to you."

"To us," she corrected me.

Linda leaned down to stroke the fawn whose mother had been killed by a car the day before.

"That vet asked you about your problems," she whispered softly to me as she caressed the fawn. "I don't remember any problems. Do you?"

I looked down at the fawn who desperately needed help and thought of all the other injured or orphaned wild creatures elsewhere that might, too. I certainly didn't want to dissuade another veterinarian from starting his own wildlife hospital.

"Can't say as I do," I replied.

Postscript

When this book was accepted for publication in February of 1984, I had no intention of adding any comment at the end. But several months ago something happened that changed my life forever.

I knew something was wrong when I began having difficulty in practice; dogs that I once could lift easily to an exam table seemed unusually heavy, and I started dropping instruments in surgery. Even handling wildlife patients became difficult. My reflexes seemed exaggerated, and my hands felt weak.

Despite my initial reluctance to admit something was wrong, deep down I knew I had a problem. Eventually I went to a neurologist and discovered I had a motor neuron disease, Amyotrophic Lateral Sclerosis (ALS). This paralyzing disease, usually fatal within four years, is commonly known as Lou Gehrig's Disease.

Despite the devastating consequences, ALS is still a rather obscure neurological disease and organizations like the ALS Society of America and the Muscular Dystrophy Association want patients to tell their stories. The hope is that the increased awareness will lead to further research, and someday a cure.

Besides that, though, I wanted to share with you some of my thoughts in recent months. In reflection, I realize that the times I spent helping injured wildlife were the best times of my life.

In fact, I like to think that there's a little "Dr. Wildlife" in most of us. It's that part that wants to reach out and help another living creature less fortunate than ourselves.

If you haven't awakened that spirit within yourself yet, there are many places that need your help. If wildlife is your interest, there are many projects like the one I started sprouting up all across the country.

If you like dogs and cats, there is a humane shelter in almost every town that could use help, even if it's only a few hours a week.

If you're not into animals at all, how about helping a handicapped or disadvantaged child or adult. There are thousands out there who could use a strong hand.

Thanks for sharing these thoughts with me. I hope that you liked reading *Dr. Wildlife*. I certainly enjoyed living it.

Rory C. Foster, DVM
Rhinelander Veterinary Medical Center
Rhinelander, WI 54501